Diabetes

Diabetes

The New Type 2

Virginia Valentine, CNS, BC-ADM, CDE,
June Biermann, *and* Barbara Toohey

JEREMY P. TARCHER/PENGUIN
a member of Penguin Group (USA) Inc.
New York

JEREMY P. TARCHER/PENGUIN
Published by the Penguin Group
Penguin Group (USA) Inc., 375 Hudson Street, New York, New York 10014, USA ·
Penguin Group (Canada), 90 Eglinton Avenue East, Suite 700, Toronto, Ontario
M4P 2Y3, Canada (a division of Pearson Canada Inc.) · Penguin Books Ltd,
80 Strand, London WC2R 0RL, England · Penguin Ireland, 25 St Stephen's Green,
Dublin 2, Ireland (a division of Penguin Books Ltd) · Penguin Group (Australia),
250 Camberwell Road, Camberwell, Victoria 3124, Australia (a division of
Pearson Australia Group Pty Ltd) · Penguin Books India Pvt Ltd, 11 Community Centre,
Panchsheel Park, New Delhi–110 017, India · Penguin Group (NZ), 67 Apollo Drive,
Rosedale, North Shore 0632, New Zealand (a division of Pearson New Zealand Ltd) ·
Penguin Books (South Africa) (Pty) Ltd, 24 Sturdee Avenue,
Rosebank, Johannesburg 2196, South Africa

Penguin Books Ltd, Registered Offices: 80 Strand, London WC2R 0RL, England

Most Tarcher/Penguin books are available at special quantity discounts for bulk purchase for sales promotions,
premiums, fund-raising, and educational needs. Special books or book excerpts also can be created to fit specific
needs. For details, write Penguin Group (USA) Inc. Special Markets, 375 Hudson Street, New York, NY 10014.

Library of Congress Cataloging-in-Publication Data

Valentine, Virginia.
Diabetes : the new type 2 / Virginia Valentine, June Biermann, and Barbara Toohey.
p.   cm.
Includes index.
"Previously published as Diabetes Type 2 and What to Do."
ISBN 978-1-58542-670-6
1. Non-insulin-dependent diabetes—Popular works.   I. Biermann, June.   II. Toohey, Barbara.   III. Title.
RC662.18.V35   2008   2008025911
616.4'62—dc22

Printed in the United States of America
1   3   5   7   9   10   8   6   4   2

BOOK DESIGN BY TANYA MAIBORODA

*I dedicate this book to my late mother, Myrna Valentine,
who was a type 2 diabetic and the epitome of what every nurse
should be; to my late father, Jay Valentine, a truly nice man;
to my daughter, Melanie, who has type 2 diabetes and who I
hope will grow up in a world without suffering from diabetes;
and to the world's best husband, John McLaughlin.*

—V.V.

*Dedicated to diabetes visionary Michael Reynolds for his wit and
perspicacity, but most of all for his enduring friendship.*

—J.B. and B.T.

Contents

Foreword

IT IS DIFFICULT TO OPEN A MAGAZINE OR A NEWSPAPER without reading that rates of obesity and diabetes are on the rise in the United States and throughout the world. Yet when diabetes is diagnosed in an individual, the facts and figures about the epidemic recede and it becomes a deeply felt, personal issue. Because of its genetic nature, many who develop type 2 diabetes have already seen family members struggle with it, some succumbing to its devastating (but now often preventable) complications. In addition, diabetes, perhaps more than any other chronic disease, conjures up feelings of guilt: guilt for being overweight or for being physically unfit; guilt for staying in denial just a little too long; and for many, worst of all, the guilt that diabetes has been passed on to the next generation.

Much of what is written about diabetes lacks connection with the true feelings experienced by people who have diabetes. When I completed my fellowship in endocrinology, in the late 1980s, I came across a book titled *The Diabetic Woman* by Lois Jovanovic, June Biermann, and Barbara Toohey. I have intense admiration for these woman, whose book is the first I'd ever read that taught me the human side to having diabetes. Now, two of those three authors, June and Barbara, have teamed up with Virginia Valentine, diabetes expert and a person with diabetes, to create an essential guide for dealing with type 2 diabetes. Their unique voices and easily readable style, along with practical advice and engaging patient stories, create a narrative that relates to the person with diabetes. This team is able to take the overwhelming facts and figures about diabetes and turn them into a recipe for daily life.

Everyone with diabetes, whether newly diagnosed or a long-term veteran, will benefit from reading *Diabetes: The New Type 2*. So, too, will family and friends whose lives are also touched by the disease. The good news is that this book, providing caring guidance from three special women, can help people with type 2 diabetes live long and healthy lives, free of complications. All it takes is a commitment to health and a willingness to learn. That and three wise women named June, Barbara, and Virginia, who can help you find a way to reach your goals.

—Anne L. Peters, M.D., CDE
Director, USC Clinical Diabetes Programs
Professor, USC Keck School of Medicine

How to Use This Book

Three for the Road to Understanding
Type 2 Diabetes

YOU ARE ABOUT TO GET ACQUAINTED WITH US AND OUR modus operandi in this book, but here's a hint of things to come.

June and Barbara have labored as a team over lo these many years, writing on many and varied topics, but primarily on matters diabetic. They continue in this collaborative mode while batting diabetes problems and solutions back and forth with Virginia.

Virginia is widely considered a learned diabetes health-care professional because that's what she is, and she has all the requisite initials after her name—as well as the national and international speaking appearances—to prove it. Also, as you will soon notice, she is by nature an indomitable spirit raiser with a sense of humor that defies depression.

So now that you know where we're coming from, let's get going.

Introduction

The Worst of Times, The Best of Times

To PARAPHRASE *A TALE OF TWO CITIES*, WE'VE BEEN THROUGH the worst of times and the best of times for type 2 diabetes.

The Worst of Times

Back in the dark ages of diabetes, when June was diagnosed, nobody really understood diabetes—and that included many doctors. June was over forty when she was told she had type 2. She was given the standard treatment for type 2 in those days, which was a casual "watch your diet, cut out sweets, lose a few pounds, get a little more exercise, and you'll be just fine." June was a person who had always been on the verge of being *under*weight, who was careful about following a healthful diet and never cared for sweets, and who was a serious walker and bike rider. Even so, she tried to follow the doctor's advice. The result was she lost weight—actually almost wasted away—and eventually had to be put on insulin to help her gain some sorely needed pounds.

From this you've probably guessed that despite her age category June turned out to have type 1 diabetes. She was insulin-deficient, meaning her body didn't produce enough insulin. She was not a type 2 like you, whose body produces plenty of insulin but can't use it effectively. More about this later, but suffice it to say that back then, many people like June had to suffer through periods of misdiagnosis.

The Best of Times

Gradually, health professionals learned about type 1 and type 2 diabetes and the profound differences between them. Consequently, more and more physicians and nurses and dietitians went into the field to help affected people know what kind of diabetes they had and how to appropriately care for it in order to live a long and happy life. And as pharmaceutical companies came to realize that there was a growing market for products and devices to help keep diabetes in good control, they became willing to invest heavily in the research and development of these products and devices. Things were clearly getting better for diabetics.

The Worst of Times and the Best of Times

But no one could call a period like the one we're in now as a total best of times. Growing numbers of people in the United States have diagnosed cases of diabetes, and untold others are running around *un*diagnosed, while diabetes, silently and slowly but surely, wreaks physical havoc on them.

Another aspect of diabetes is turning out to be the worst of the worst, as children and young people are developing type 2 diabetes as never before. But take heart. We're not going to let diabetes sneak up on us as it has in the past. Everyone is becoming more aware of diabetes and is determined to do something about it now. We know it can and will happen. In fact, one of the movers and shakers in making things happen in type 2 diabetes is our collaborator, Virginia Valentine.

We were privileged to find her through our friend, the eminent endocrinologist Lois Jovanovic, M.D., with whom we collaborated on *The Diabetic Woman.* We wrote to tell her we thought there really needed to be a book strictly devoted to type 2 diabetes, and to ask if she would be interested in collaborating with us on it. Dr. Jovanovic was quick to respond that she agreed such a book needed to be written, but that it would be a thousand times more meaningful if our collaborator had type 2 diabetes. For that reason, she suggested someone other than herself, since she's a type 1. Her recommendation was a person whom she described as "a type 2 who uses her condition to motivate and win the hearts and minds of other type 2s. She has won the Educator of the Year Award for the state of Oklahoma and the national award from the American Association of Diabetes Educators. She is witty, clever, and smart, too." She was referring to Virginia Valentine, CNS, CDE, who was at that time the clinical nurse specialist for diabetes at the University of New Mexico Medical Center in Albuquerque, and is currently the CEO of Diabetes Network, as well as clinical associate faculty at the University of New Mexico College of Nursing and School of Medicine.

As we quickly learned, and as you will see in this book, everything Dr. Jovanovic said about Virginia proved to be true—and then some! She tells type 2 like it is because she lives it like it is and has been doing so for the last twenty-eight years. Trust us you can trust her.

—*June Biermann and Barbara Toohey*

I Don't Have a Character Flaw and Neither Do You!

I have had type 2 diabetes for twenty-eight years. I was diagnosed at age thirty, which, as most textbooks will tell you, is much too young to get this type of diabetes. In 1980 I was an anomaly, and my doctor thought I had "juvenile" diabetes. Sadly, we now see type 2 diabetes way too often in young people, even children.

Most people, when they're diagnosed with diabetes, ask, "Why me, Lord?" But since there was so much history of diabetes on both sides of my family, I guess I always knew that eventually I would get it. My question was, "Why now, Lord?" I wasn't supposed to get diabetes until after age forty. Although I felt a little cheated at getting it at such an early age, I wasn't all that worried because my paternal grandfather, who had diabetes, lived to be almost eighty, and my mother's aunts and cousins with diabetes didn't have any of the terrible complications that I was to see later when I went to work in the field of diabetes.

After several years in college as an art and advertising major, I chose to go into nursing when I realized that I wanted to do something that had a more significant impact on people. My mother was a nurse, but I had not previously considered that profession because I thought all nurses had to be as smart as she was—and I felt that left me out.

Then the summer after my sophomore year in college, I didn't have a summer job. Mothers can't stand it if they see you sleeping late and frittering away your time, so my mom made me come to the hospital to help out in the nursery. I was petrified of handling those little babies, but that summer I did discover two things that I'd not previously known or appreciated: (1) most nurses were not as smart as my mom (which is not a put-down of nurses but praise for my mom, who was a genius), and therefore I could probably handle the schooling; and (2) the essence of nursing is not shots and bedpans, but bringing out the inner healing reserves of people. That was the part of the job I really liked. I decided I would take college algebra and chemistry as a personal test to see if I could survive. I figured if I could live through those courses, I'd be able to manage nursing school. I could and I did.

In nursing school I discovered for myself something my mother had already told me: medical patients are much more interesting than surgical patients. Medical service is where they put the older patients with chronic diseases. Among health professionals, the job of caring for patients with chronic diseases is not considered as glamorous as surgery, but I found the work much more rewarding and exciting. In medical service you get to know your patients and develop meaningful relationships with them.

A few years after graduating with a baccalaureate degree in nursing from Central State University in Oklahoma, I became pregnant with my first (and last!) baby. They told me I had gestational diabetes—that's the kind of diabetes that sometimes emerges during a pregnancy and then goes away after the baby is delivered. In 1976, most centers were not screening for gestational diabetes on a routine basis, but I was under the care of the university faculty, and they were checking for this. Although they recognized what it was, they didn't know much about treating it. Mainly what they did was to tell me to watch my sugar intake. (Sound familiar?) I followed their limited instructions, except I didn't eat as many calories as they suggested. And still I had a twelve-pound baby at full term. (In the past, overweight babies were typical for women with diabetes.) She was beautiful, twenty-five inches long, with thick, dark, curly hair. She made all the other babies in the nursery look anemic.

Then, just as the textbooks tell you, five years later I was diagnosed with diabetes. At the time, I was in graduate school at the University of Oklahoma College of Nursing specializing in chronic disease, and my husband and I were in the process of getting a divorce. (Could it be that I was under stress?) Since I was overweight and had very high blood sugar levels, my doctor immediately put me on insulin. I was on insulin for about a year before I decided to start figuring things out for myself. I lost fifty pounds and got off insulin and remained diet controlled for the next eight years. Eighteen years ago, I had to go on oral hypoglycemic agents (pills) to control my blood sugar, and weight control is a never-ending battle for me.

In 1982, when I attended a diabetes management training program in New York with Dr. Lois Jovanovic, I learned that women with diabetes didn't have to have twelve-pound babies. To my sorrow, I also learned that my child would be at a greatly increased risk for type 2 diabetes herself, not only because I had type 2 diabetes, but because she had developed increased fat cells during gestation. (I think motherhood should be renamed guilthood.)

Melanie, now in her thirties and overweight, has had diabetes since her early twenties. She is a great kid who works hard to maintain good diabetes control. Hopefully, we will have an answer for her children so that they will not experience the same fate as the rest of the family.

Since 1981 I've primarily worked in areas helping people with diabetes. I love helping people with chronic diseases because they're so downtrodden—the stepchildren of the health-care system. It's pretty amazing that these patients are treated this way when you think about it, since diabetes affects almost 10 percent of the population in America. Many people—and that includes many health professionals who should know better—treat type 2 diabetes as if it is only a punishment for being fat. The implication is that if you weren't fat you wouldn't have the disease, and therefore, it's all your own fault. I know this is true, because I've had more than one physician tell me the same. I consider it a privilege to be able to make a difference for people who have my affliction. I am now a consultant for health-care agencies and the pharmaceutical industry, and I have a business in New Mexico called Diabetes Network with my business partner Catherine Gray. We provide diabetes education and case management at our diabetes center in Albuquerque and in a large number of primary-care clinics in central New Mexico. We work with most of the insurance companies in the area and the largest health-care system in the state, which takes an enlightened approach toward diabetes. They have prioritized diabetes control in their system and have been able to make a big difference for people with diabetes in their care.

That's why my message in this book is: diabetes is not a character flaw! If you believe that you have diabetes because you're fat, ask yourself these questions: why are there so many people out there fatter than you who don't have diabetes? Why do half the members of the Pima tribe of American Indians in Arizona have type 2 diabetes? Why do people with diabetes have parents and grandparents who also have diabetes?

I'll answer these questions for you. Type 2 diabetes in overweight people is a disorder in the way food is metabolized (converted to energy) and used in the body. Yes, lifestyle does affect diabetes, but when you look at the research reports on type 2, you see that the origin is in the genes you're born with. It is genetically determined, just like the color of your eyes. (And nobody calls your blue or brown eyes a character flaw.)

Probably in the next ten years we'll see treatments directed toward the correction of these metabolic errors. What we have to do in the meantime is learn to live with the disease in such a way that we can stay healthy and participate fully in our lives. For me, participating fully in life means helping my patients and living in Albuquerque with the world's greatest husband and daughter. To do that I have to constantly work at diabetes management myself. The major challenge for me is to stay on a healthy diet and get some exercise every day.

The American Diabetes Association once had a mission: "a world without diabetes." When I first saw that statement, I tried to picture a world without diabetes, and I couldn't stretch my imagination to visualize such a thing. Maybe the end of type 1 diabetes can be achieved, but I can't bring myself to even dream of a world without type 2. I have to alter that phrase into "a world without suffering from diabetes." In my view, that means helping people keep their blood sugar in the near-normal range so they don't suffer the terrible, disabling complications of diabetes. It also means helping people make the necessary lifestyle changes for diabetes management without suffering—giving them common-sense approaches tailored to the individual. Above all, I want to keep them from feeling blamed for the disease they inherited.

For me, a world without suffering from diabetes is available right now, not something we have to wait for until a far-distant day. My reason for writing this book is to show you how, together, we can achieve this new kind of world for people with type 2 diabetes.

—*Virginia Valentine, CNS, BC-ADM, CDE*

NOTE FOR THOSE WITH A CHILD WHO IS DEVELOPING, OR IS AT RISK OF DEVELOPING, TYPE 2 DIABETES

It's only understandable that you want to learn about children's type 2 diabetes and you want to learn it *right now*. We have that information for you. You will find it starting on page 244 but it might be a good idea for you to first read all the general information on type 2 that comes in the beginning of the book. That way, you'll have a solid base of knowledge to build on. But if you can't contain yourself, go ahead and read the children's section, then come back to the beginning and start over. It really doesn't matter where or when or how you get your information, the important thing is to get it—and act on it.

1

Type 2 Diabetes

What Is This Thing Called Diabetes?

JUNE DESCRIBES A SCIENTIFIC DEFINITION AS "A TERM YOU don't understand explained in words you don't understand." Nowhere is this more true than in diabetes. When you're first diagnosed and have no idea of what diabetes is and how it's going to affect your life, *wham!* you're hit with a whole bunch of unfamiliar terms for your type of diabetes.

We don't want to start this book with a lot of confusing lingo. On the contrary, our goal is to use what we might call "beginner's language" so you can ease into a diabetes vocabulary that will serve you well over the years and allow you to communicate effectively with diabetes health-care professionals (physicians, nurses, dietitians), allowing them to communicate effectively with you. Here goes your first vocabulary lesson.

First off, what is diabetes? It is a chronic (meaning it's for the rest of your life, or at least until they find a cure) physical problem that causes you to have too much sugar in your blood. Diabetes health-care professionals often call the sugar in your blood "glucose," a more specific (and scientific) term. The medical term for high blood sugar is hyperglycemia ("hyper" in this case means too much, and "glycemia" refers to glucose in the blood). Low blood sugar is called hypoglycemia ("hypo" means too little). Euglycemia, a term used less often than the other two, might be called Goldilocks blood sugar because it's just right—not too high and not too low; in other words, it's normal blood sugar, which is what people without diabetes have. The word "euglycemia" has the same prefix as euphoria—eu: a feeling of happiness and well-being. And euphoria is exactly what you'll feel when you get your hyperglycemia down to euglycemia. The goal of all the advice and counsel in this book is simply to move you into that ideal realm of normal blood sugar.

The American Diabetes Association defines diabetes as "a disease in which the body does not produce or respond to insulin (a hormone produced by the pancreas). Without insulin your body cannot properly convert the food you eat into energy." They go on to point out that diabetes is actually a general term for a number of separate but related disorders. "These disorders fall into two main categories: type 1 and type 2." And since you're reading this book, we're assuming you're a type 2.

What is the difference between these two types of diabetes? That was clarified in guidelines announced in June 1997 (the old ones dated from 1979) and updated every year since by an Expert Committee convened by the American Diabetes Association. Besides redefining the categories of diabetes, the Expert Committee converted the former Roman numerals into Arabic numerals to avoid confusion. (Virginia guesses they must have thought people would read the Roman numerals wrong and think they had type 11, or eleven, diabetes.) All the older books still use type I and type II, but now you know better—and you'll know when you're reading an older, possibly outdated, book. You may still see in some books—and hear from some diabetes health-care people—some of the now outmoded terms for type 2, such as maturity-onset, non-insulin-dependent, or even NIDDM—non-insulin-dependent diabetes mellitus. (There's a term we won't miss.)

Here are the current ADA definitions of type 1 and type 2 diabetes (it pays to know the difference in case you haven't been correctly diagnosed):

In type 1 diabetes your body destroys the cells in the pancreas that produce insulin, usually leading to a total failure to produce insulin. It typically starts in children or young adults who are slim, but it can start at any age. It afflicts about 1 to 1 1/2 million Americans. In type 2 diabetes the body cannot use insulin properly and sometimes—especially if you've had diabetes for a long time—it doesn't produce enough insulin. It used to occur almost exclusively in people over forty-five and overweight, among other factors. In 2007, about 14 million Americans had been diagnosed and another 6 million (according to the American Diabetes Association—Diabetes.org) remained undiagnosed with type 2 diabetes.

TOTAL: 20.8 million children and adults—7.0 percent of the population—have diabetes.

DIAGNOSED: 14.6 million people

UNDIAGNOSED: 6.2 million people

PREDIABETES: 54 million people

In 2005, 1.5 million cases of diabetes (both type 1 and type 2) were diagnosed in people age twenty and older.

Total Prevalence of Diabetes

UNDER TWENTY YEARS OF AGE: Of all people in this age group, 176,500, or 0.22 percent, have diabetes. About one in every four hundred to six hundred children and adolescents has type 1 diabetes.

Two million adolescents (or one in six overweight adolescents) ages twelve to nineteen have prediabetes.

Although type 2 diabetes can occur in youth, the nationally representative data that would be needed to monitor diabetes trends in youth by type are not available. Clinically based reports and regional studies suggest that type 2 diabetes, although still rare, is being diagnosed more frequently in children and adolescents, particularly in American Indians, African-Americans, and Hispanic/Latino Americans.

AGE TWENTY YEARS OR OLDER: Of all people in this age group, 20.6 million, or 9.6 percent, have diabetes.

AGE SIXTY YEARS OR OLDER: Of all people in this age group, 10.3 million, or 20.9 percent, have diabetes.

MEN: Of all men age twenty years or older, 10.9 million, or 10.5 percent, have diabetes, although nearly one-third of them do not know it.

WOMEN: Of all women age twenty years or older, 9.7 million, or 8.8 percent, have diabetes, although nearly one-third of them do not know it. The prevalence of diabetes is at least two to four times higher among non-Hispanic black, Hispanic/Latino American, American Indian, and Asian/Pacific Islander women than among non-Hispanic white women.

And the dismal type 2 diabetes statistical beat goes on. A study in the September 2000 issue of the journal *Diabetes Care* reported that from 1990 to 1998 the incidence of diabetes increased at an unprecedented rate. An alarming—and startling—development was that there was an increase of 76 percent in diabetes cases among people in their thirties. In days gone by, type 2 diabetes usually developed two or more decades later in life. Now even more alarming and startling is the fact that children and young people are developing type 2. Recent studies report as many as 45 percent of children diagnosed with diabetes are type 2s.

Dr. Frank Vinicor of the Centers for Disease Control and Prevention predicts that "it's going to get considerably worse in the future." Why? Experts in the field say the blame is right in front of our noses: the television and computer screens that encourage people of all ages to sit for hours literally on end. This sedentarianism with the concomitant lack of exercise and the ever-present temptation of high-calorie snacks has created an almost epidemic rise in obesity. Although certainly not all overweight people develop diabetes, the risk factor for diabetes does increase along with the excess pounds.

But enough of dismal statistics and predictions and back to the underlying question of what is this thing called diabetes that is burgeoning at such an unheard-of rate?

As we said before, in both types of diabetes the basic problem is that without treatment there is too much sugar in the blood. In this first chapter we'll ask Virginia to interpret and amplify these definitions—and to explain how and why you develop diabetes and in what direction you should go with your diabetes therapy to correct your abnormally high blood sugar.

—*June and Barbara*

Definitions of Diabetes

June and Barbara: Virginia, how do you explain to your patients the meaning of type 2 diabetes and how they fit into the picture?

Virginia: I think this new classification system is much clearer than the one we used to use. Of course, there are variations with the type 1 and type 2 groups. The variations could explain why most people get type 1 diabetes before the age of twenty, and then some, like June, get it later in life. You can still differentiate type 1s from the 2s by the amount of insulin their bodies make. You can either do a C-peptide test (this indicates the amount of insulin being made by your pancreas), or you can use the less expensive alternative: just take a look at your body shape. It takes insulin to store fat. By looking at most of us who have type 2 diabetes, you can see that they make plenty of insulin. You can't get "fluffy" without insulin. I have had a lifelong battle with obesity and in the last five and a half years have reached a new level of weight that I haven't seen since high school. June, on the other hand, has a hard time storing fat, and without insulin, she would rapidly drop weight. Type 1s usually have an absolute insulin deficiency that could be caused either by an autoimmune process (the immune system gets confused and mistakenly destroys its own insulin-making cells called "beta cells" in the islets of Langerhans located in the pancreas) or by an idiopathic (of unknown cause) process.

We type 2 people, on the other hand, have what's called insulin resistance. This means the basic problem is the muscle cells' resistance to our own insulin, so our insulin can't move glucose into our other cells. Our glucose has no place to go, so our blood sugar keeps getting higher and higher. This alerts the pancreas to start making extra insulin to take care of the glucose. Eventually insulin-making cells grow so weary of trying to produce enough insulin that they just give up, leaving you with what we unscientifically—but accurately—call "pancreatic poop-out." In recent years we have learned about new hormones that are critical to this complex process of converting food into fuel. First, we make a hormone in the beta cell called amylin. This hormone is like insulin's long-lost brother. It helps insulin do its job by telling the liver to quit making too much extra glucose and slowing the stomach from releasing food too fast, and helps you feel satisfied so you eat less. Since people with type 1 have few beta cells, they are both insulin and amylin deficient. Many people with type 2 diabetes who require insulin may also be amylin deficient. Fortunately, we now have a synthetic amylin, called Symlin, to help folks with diabetes with improving after-meal glucose levels.

So if you have type 2 you are considered relatively insulin deficient. No, that doesn't mean your relatives are insulin deficient. It is important to realize that people with type 2 are making insulin, but just not enough to overcome their resistance and keep their blood sugar normal.

June and Barbara: How do you know the type 2s are still making some insulin of their own?

Virginia: We know because they rarely, if ever, go into diabetic coma, or, as we say in medical circles, diabetic ketoacidosis (often abbreviated DKA). DKA is caused by extremely high blood sugars from lack of insulin. The type 2s are protected from DKA because they still make some insulin, at least enough so that some glucose can get into their cells and prevent the body from sending out the message that it's starving. That message tells the body to start breaking down fat and converting it to glucose. When this happens, the conversion of fat and protein to glucose leaves a waste product called ketones. These are acid products that raise the acid level in the body. When your acid-base balance is upset, your normal metabolic processes cannot work. This is a serious medical crisis that calls for immediate hospitalization. Typically, people with type 1 diabetes will report that, especially at times of stress from illness, they've had bouts of DKA. But it is unusual for an adult type 2 to experience DKA, and if it does happen, it's usually at a time of extreme stress, such as a surgery.

June and Barbara: That's certainly a piece of welcome news. But we've heard there's something similar to DKA that type 2s *can* develop. Strangely enough we read about this in the novel *At Home in Mitford*, by Jan Karon. It's the story of Father Tim, an Episcopalian rector who has type 2 diabetes and, as a result of overextending himself in service to his parishioners, winds up in the hospital in nonketotic hyperglycemic coma. Could you tell us what that is?

Virginia: It's also known as hyperosmolar coma and is an acute medical emergency that sometimes affects type 2s. This happens when blood sugars become inordinately high (symptoms of the hyperosmolar state are dehydration, drowsiness, and confusion). Loss of consciousness and, in some cases, death can occur. The person must be treated in a hospital with fluid replacement and insulin. Usually when a type 2 has ketones in the urine they are the "ketones of starvation," which means they are produced when you are running low on glucose and it is a way for your body to convert stored energy (fat) into fuel for your brain. People trying to lose weight on very low-carbohydrate diets will see ketones in urine (more about this in the section on diets).

June and Barbara: Now that we've given you these dire warnings about ketones, we should mention that there are times when ketones are welcome. These are when you're trying to lose weight and are following a low-carbohydrate diet. They indicate that you are burning fat. These ketones are what the author and controversial diet "guru" Dr. Richard K. Bernstein calls "benign ketones," meaning they don't lead to DKA. You'll read more about this in the section on the low-carbohydrate, high-protein diet on page 180.

Not only have the definitions of diabetes been revised, but also the methods of diagnosis. What can you tell us about this?

Virginia: Yes, the other big news from the new classification system is the blood sugar level number for diagnosing diabetes. If you have a fasting blood sugar (before breakfast) of over 126 mg/dl, you are now considered diabetic. (**Note:** Blood sugar numbers refer to milligrams [mg] of glucose per deciliter [dl] of blood. We often omit the mg/dl after the number in this book.) In the old diagnosis system, you weren't classified as having diabetes until your fasting blood sugar was over 140 mg/dl. Many people already had the complications of diabetes (nerve, eye, and kidney damage) when their fasting level had reached 140.

The other problem with the old system was that you weren't considered to have diabetes until your blood sugar was over 200 two hours after a glucose challenge. A glucose challenge could be a glucose drink designed to diagnose diabetes, or it could be the "IHOP challenge." We often send folks out for pancakes and juice and then do a two-hour glucose test. That will challenge your pancreas as well as a glucose drink. It turns out when your post glucose challenge glucose is 200, your fasting glucose is about 125. By diagnosing at or above 126, people can treat their blood glucose levels earlier and avoid many of the complications.

Another improvement is the recommendation for regular screening of the general population for diabetes. This is a real departure from previous standards. The U.S. Centers for Disease Control estimates that there are 16 million people with diabetes, but one-third don't know they have it. (Funny how the CDC should know, but the people who have it don't.) Because there are so many undiagnosed people out there, they now recommend screening all people over forty-five years of age every three years.

June and Barbara: It's high time somebody woke up to the fact that much of the problem with the destructive consequences of undiagnosed diabetes can be prevented. June was diagnosed with a blood sugar of 425 (normal is about 70 to 100), and we're always hearing of those who only find out about their diabetes after their high sugars have given them significant symptoms of complications because they've already had the disease for many years.

Can you tell us how type 2 diabetes slowly develops over the years and how it affects your body?

Virginia: There are three problems that lead to type 2. We'll take them in the order they most often occur, although they don't necessarily develop in such a clear-cut way.

Insulin Resistance and Hyperinsulinemia (Too Much Insulin)

In type 2 diabetes the insulin produced by your pancreas does not work as it should because over the years your body cells have become resistant to it. They don't accept it as they once did. (Scientists aren't sure yet why this happens.) The cells in your body have receptors that, if working properly, accept the insulin. This coupling triggers a chain of events that open the cells to accept glucose (the sugar your body uses as fuel). If muscle cells don't use the glucose, it will be stored as fat.

When your body notices that your insulin isn't working to move glucose into the cells, it gets busy and makes more insulin. You then develop what we call hyperinsulinemia, or too much insulin in your blood. Insulin is a powerful fat-generating hormone. This extra insulin, then, causes you to store fat and to be very hungry. By eating more to satisfy your insulin-induced hunger, you add even more weight. The extra fat caused by too much insulin and too much eating further increases your insulin resistance. Putting the two together, you now have the initial insulin resistance caused by type 2 diabetes plus the additional insulin resistance caused by being overweight—a vicious cycle if ever there was one.

Inadequate Insulin Production

Now we come to the second of the three problems that cause type 2 diabetes. So far the story is that you started many, many years before with insulin resistance. This caused your body to make extra insulin to try to move the glucose into your cells so that your blood glucose would stay normal. You probably had a weight problem to begin with and gained more weight over the years because of the extra insulin. When, then, did you actually become a person with diabetes? When your body could no longer make enough extra insulin to compensate for the resistance. Let me make it clear that you're not really deficient in insulin—you're making way over the normal amount but what you make is not enough, considering your needs, to keep your blood glucose at the normal level, so you end up with high blood glucose. In other words, you have diabetes.

Excess Liver Metabolism

Now you're insulin resistant, without enough insulin even though you're still making a whole bunch of it, and your blood glucose is higher in the morning than it was when you went to bed. The explanation for this is that you have developed what we call excess liver glucose production. That's right, just when you thought things couldn't get worse, your liver gets into the act. When you haven't eaten in quite a few hours (since supper), your liver thinks it needs to start giving back some of the stored-up glucose for this kind of emergency. The liver either releases stored glucose or it can convert protein into glucose. When your liver starts kicking in after a six- or eight-hour fast, because your insulin resistance keeps the glucose from getting into the cells, the liver pours in extra glucose, so you wake up with terribly high blood sugar, even though it was normal when you went to bed.

Now, it turns out, we have some additional problems to add to the mix. The person with type 2 diabetes is becoming amylin deficient along with insulin resistance. Remember, amylin is a hormone made in the beta cell along with insulin and it helps keep the liver in check and slow the amount of fuel added to blood glucose by slowing stomach emptying and improving your feeling of satiety (feeling full). Another hormone may play an even bigger part in this play. A gut hormone called GLP-1 is made in the intestines when you eat and it helps in four ways:

1. GLP-1 stimulates the beta cell to increase its insulin production and it makes insulin in a more normal way. Also, by stimulating insulin production from the beta cell, you will also get an increase in amylin.
2. It turns down the glucose production from the liver.
3. The hormone slows emptying from the stomach.
4. It increases satiety so you eat less.

To sum up, since you have a resistance to insulin, your cells can't make use of the insulin as they should. Your pancreas is making a lot of insulin, but it's still not enough to overcome your resistance. And your liver doesn't understand why the glucose it's releasing isn't getting into your cells, so it does the only thing it knows how to do: it keeps producing more and more glucose, and that makes your blood sugar go higher and higher. Your "helper" hormone GLP-1 is diminished and that contributes to decreased insulin, especially "first phase" insulin, which is the first squirt of insulin that is made normally. That's how diabetes develops and keeps getting worse until you get proper treatment to bring it under control.

June and Barbara: To help us better understand all this, could you tell us a typical story of how one individual's type 2 diabetes might have developed over the years? Then each of our readers can visualize what probably happened to bring on his or her diabetes.

Virginia: Yes, I can easily trace for you the physiological history of a typical case of type 2 diabetes. Let's call the heroine of our story Helen. We'll say that she's fifty-five years old, overweight, feeling sluggish, has dry, itchy skin, is subject to frequent slow-healing infections, and has tingling in her toes. She makes a doctor's appointment, is examined and tested, and is diagnosed with type 2 diabetes. (These are typical symptoms, but sometimes there are absolutely no signs that would cue the person to go to the doctor.)

HELEN'S STORY

Let's go back ten to twenty years ago, when Helen develops the problem of insulin resistance (she is not aware of this, of course). To overcome this resistance, her body starts making extra insulin to try to get the glucose from her food into the cells, where it can be used as fuel. The extra insulin does keep her blood sugars normal, and therefore she is still nondiabetic. The extra insulin also causes her to gain weight, because it makes her store as fat a higher percentage of the food she eats. Soon she'll refer to herself as the type of person who can gain five pounds just smelling a plate of brownies—and she almost can! She is also becoming deficient in her helper hormone GLP-1, and that is probably contributing to her hunger.

After a few years, the excessive insulin she is making to compensate for her resistance is no longer enough. Now her type 2 pancreas starts losing its ability to produce the huge amounts of insulin she needs. Normally, when a person starts eating a meal, the body sends out a little squirt of insulin within minutes. This is called the first-phase insulin response. You can control your blood sugar a lot better if you have insulin right there at the door to meet the food than if you have to conquer a high blood sugar after the meal. Helen's body now refuses to send out enough insulin to cover that first-phase insulin response.

Look at the two-part diagram in Figure 1.1. The first part shows how the normal pancreas sends out a small amount of insulin at the beginning of a meal, followed by a second-phase response that sends

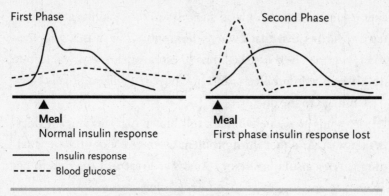

Figure 1.1 • **Insulin Response to a Meal**

out a larger amount of insulin to keep the blood sugar from going up after the finish of the meal. The second bump of insulin prevents blood sugar from going up more than 20 or 40 points (or mg/dl). We use the term points for simplification. Thus, 20 points would be 20 mg/dl and 40 points would be 40 mg/dl. In other words, the person without diabetes who starts out with a blood sugar before meals of 70 or 80 may go up after the meal to 110 or 120. It's not normal to have wide swings in blood sugars throughout the day.

The second part shows what happens to blood sugar levels when you lose the first-phase insulin response. The blood sugar spikes up way above normal levels until the second phase kicks in.

So without her first-phase insulin response, Helen is now beginning to cross over into diabetes territory. As her blood sugars climb, they tend to stay up because it takes more insulin to conquer a high than to maintain a normal blood sugar. One year Helen's fasting blood sugar might be in the 90s and after meals in the 130s to 140s. A couple of Thanksgiving and Christmas celebrations later, she'll get fasting readings running 100 to 110 and get up to 150 to 160 after meals. It's something that just sneaks up on you little by little.

The phenomenon in which Helen's insulin doesn't work as well to conquer high sugars as it does to handle normal ones is called glucose toxicity. Blood sugar levels of 150 to 180 are considered toxic, because that's where the trouble that causes complications begins. These are the kinds of blood sugars that will lead to the fatigue, skin problems, and tinglings that will eventually cause Helen to go to the doctor.

Helen is now a person with full-blown diabetes, but she doesn't know it. And that third problem we talked about before is setting in. Her insulin resistance is now so great that the cells in her liver that are supposed to notice all that insulin in her bloodstream have totally lost their ability to detect it. In the middle of the night after four or five hours of nothing to eat, her liver's job is to start putting glucose into her bloodstream as her blood sugar drops. The liver is a storage tank of fuel so that we never run out, even when we don't eat. Helen's liver, since it can't detect the presence of insulin in her bloodstream (its signal that there's food there), goes berserk. It pours out lots and lots of glucose. Helen gets excessive liver glucose production and delivery in the night, so she gets up in the morning with high blood sugar. That high morning blood sugar means she'll be high all day long, since her insulin no longer has the ability to bring down high blood sugars. When she finally goes to the doctor and has a blood sugar test, she'll find out why she doesn't feel well anymore.

"Thrifty" Genes

June and Barbara: Our next logical question for you is why do some over-forty-five and overweight people get diabetes, while others go on blithely, getting even more and more overweight, but they never develop diabetes. What factors make the difference?

Virginia: Type 2 is a genetic disease that runs in families. It is much more hereditary than type 1. In studies of identical twins, in cases where one twin gets type 1 diabetes, 40 percent to 50 percent of the identical siblings get the disease; when one twin gets type 2, 90 percent of the identical siblings develop diabetes.

June and Barbara: In your introduction, Virginia, you mentioned that not only is there a type 2 diabetes gene, but also another genetic disorder that contributes to type 2. We understand that this second disorder has to do with the way food is metabolized (converted to energy) and accounts for the way being overweight and getting diabetes go together (and they do go together because about 90 percent of type 2s are overweight). Can you describe the metabolic error that causes the initial weight problem of most type 2s, a problem that is later made worse by excess insulin production?

Virginia: To understand this disorder we have to go back to our origins in this country—to the tribes of American Indians who were here in the first place. I said that between 6 percent and 10 percent of the U.S. population has diabetes, but that's the overall figure. In American Indians, Hispanics, and African-Americans, the incidence of diabetes is more than double that of those of us of European descent. Diabetes favors minorities, and the most favored of all are our American Indian citizens.

American Indians are two to three times more likely to get diabetes than Anglos. The professionals who work with the Indian Health Service explain this extraordinary rate of diabetes with the "thrifty gene" theory. This theory starts with the plight of the indigenous peoples a few thousand years ago. Imagine yourself living in America as a Zuni or a Sioux. Your life is one of strenuous hard work, and starvation is a major cause of death. Some persons evolve a metabolism that is very efficient and can "store" a higher percentage of food than other people. These are the people who will live through the winter, because they use less of their food for energy and store more of what they eat for times of famine. These are the ones who reproduce and pass on their lifesaving metabolism.

June and Barbara: That doesn't sound like a metabolic error, but more like a metabolic advantage.

Virginia: Then was then and now is now. The advantage changes into a disadvantage when you take people into the twenty-first century. Give people cars and a diet high in fat (fat foods are stored as fat in the body more quickly than protein or carbohydrate foods), and you have people who gain weight easily, coupled with a built-in genetic tendency toward type 2 diabetes. These people have both insulin resistance and a metabolism designed to survive famine. With a body programmed like this, it's a real challenge to overcome civilization. With this genetic double whammy, the American Indians in the United States are being devastated by diabetes. In many tribes, as many as half the adults have type 2 diabetes. Gestational diabetes (the form that emerges during pregnancy) occurs in as many as 20 percent of pregnancies, compared to 3 percent in the rest of the population. This will only perpetuate the cycle. Amputations and kidney failure are occurring in the American Indian population at rates that stagger the imagination. A couple of summers ago I visited the Hualapai tribe near the Grand Canyon in Arizona. This village of fifteen hundred people has a kidney failure rate one thousand times greater than the national average.

Recently I was in Sacaton, Arizona, and had the opportunity to meet many of the Pima people, 50 percent of whom have diabetes. Let me tell you about Joy. She is thirty-six years old and has had diabetes for three years. It's not uncommon to find Pima children eight and ten years old with type 2 diabetes. I talked with Joy about getting better control of her blood glucose levels without having to go on insulin. She's already at the maximum dose of oral agents (blood sugar–lowering pills). She was very receptive to trying a Fast Fast (carbohydrate-restricted diet; see Chapter 4) for a few days and then working on her diet, although I must tell you she was already doing most things right.

She told me she does not allow any cookies or chips in her house and wants to make sure her children eat right so that they don't get diabetes. That made me very sad, because it is not chips and cookies that are going to give her children diabetes. Of course, no one needs chips and cookies (except in rare emergencies), but we must not blame the disease on the patient. Joy will help her children eat better and live longer, because they're working on low-fat and high-fiber eating patterns.

For the sake of Joy's and all the Pima children, I hope we will find the answer to prevent and cure this disease. All the Pima people I met are very concerned about their health and the well-being of their families. It's very disturbing to see the level of devastation that diabetes is causing in these lovely people.

Who Gets Diabetes?

June and Barbara: The Diabetes Prevention Program for type 2 diabetes is a study that was designed to explore ways to prevent or delay diabetes. Did this study yield positive results?

Virginia: Yes. In this study they enrolled people with impaired glucose tolerance, sometimes called "borderline" diabetes. They assigned them to either the control group (do nothing), the group receiving metformin (trade name is Glucophage) and a third group receiving "intensive lifestyle change" (makes me sweat to think about it). After three and a half years they stopped the study early because the results were so dramatic. They found that if you do nothing, about 10 percent–11 percent proceed to develop diabetes. The metformin group, though, was 30 percent less likely to develop diabetes. The most interesting finding is that the diet and exercise group was almost 60 percent less likely to progress to diabetes. The diet and exercise program was called intensive, but actually the participants lost on average about fifteen pounds and exercised thirty minutes a day for five days a week, mostly by walking. These results have finally provided some hope for people on the path to diabetes. We now know that we can definitely and possibly prevent type 2 diabetes. The difficult part is getting folks to lose weight and exercise and keep it up. This study was expensive and required a large number of people to get this successful outcome. They are continuing to study the people in the trial to see how the disease progresses.

June and Barbara: We know that besides American Indians, the Hispanic population has a high incidence of type 2—about 13 percent or 14 percent. Even more appalling, we've heard that 30 percent to 40 percent of Hispanic women over age fifty-five have diabetes. Why do Hispanic people also have such a high rate of type 2 diabetes?

Virginia: This is an interesting question, because if you go back to the Spanish ancestors of today's Hispanics, you do not find an increased rate of diabetes. The Spanish explorers who came to America brought a rich cultural heritage and horses, but it seems they did not bring diabetes to America. The Hispanic people of Mexico and the Southwest often forget that their Spanish ancestors who populated the area in the 1600s did not bring any women with them. Their high rate of diabetes is a genetic heirloom from the local Indian people with whom the Spanish mingled and married. People of Hispanic descent in America are ten to fifteen times more likely to develop diabetes than the Anglo population. Most of them will get type 2 diabetes, although there are Hispanic people who have type 1.

June and Barbara: That brings us to the African-American population. Ten percent of African-Americans suffer from diabetes, and it's the third leading cause of death in their racial group. An article in the February 1991 *Diabetes Forecast* explained that the high occurrence of obesity among African-Americans contributes greatly to this. And the main reason for their high rate of obesity (60 percent of African-American women over forty-five years of age are obese) is poverty and the diet that poverty imposes on them. Thirty-four percent of African-American men and women are below the poverty line, while only about 11 percent of white men and women are. Poverty and obesity, as the article puts it, often go together. The problem is confounded because African-Americans also have "thrifty" genes.

And now, Virginia, we finally come to people like you. You have those "thrifty" genes but you're an Anglo. Where do you fit in?

Virginia: True, I'm not an American Indian, even though I was raised in Oklahoma, and I am neither Hispanic nor African-American, but I got diabetes at a young age, just as some of the populations with high rates of diabetes do. In fact, they're getting it at younger and younger ages. I have a Norwegian grandmother, and I have diabetes on both sides of my family. Lots of Northern European peoples developed the same "efficient" metabolism that allowed them to survive feast-or-famine lifestyles. In fact, type 2 diabetes is increasing in the general population of the United States at the rate of 6 percent a year.

This brings me to something I heard the other day that goes along with this discussion of how type 2 diabetes is Mother Nature's way of maintaining the species. An overweight man with type 2 diabetes named Frank came into our center. Frank had been a prisoner of war in World War II, and when we explained to him how type 2 diabetes works and why he has the problems he does, he got this sudden enlightened look on his face. "So that's why I never lost weight in the prison camp!" he exclaimed.

He went on to tell us how he had been in the camp for almost a year and was about the same weight when he came out as when he went in, while his comrades were reduced to skin and bones. He said, "Granted, I did get a little more food than my buddies did because I could speak Italian. I would go over and talk to the Italian prisoners, and they would sometimes slip me a little pasta or something. But I certainly didn't get anywhere near the kind of food I needed, and yet I hardly lost any weight at all. I always wondered about that."

This is an excellent illustration of the fact that simply decreasing calories is not the way to lose weight. A low-calorie diet alone is absolutely not going to help the person with type 2 diabetes. You see, the other aspect of being a prisoner of war was that Frank got almost no exercise, being confined to a small space.

What we're doing now with Frank is first working on having him cut down the amount of fat he's eating. But I've told him what I have to tell all people with type 2 diabetes: his chances of getting down to an ideal body weight are two—a slim chance and no chance at all. So you see, it's especially important that we set other goals for ourselves: the goals of being healthy and fit. Fit means normal levels of blood sugar, normal blood lipids (the blood fats that can cause heart disease), normal blood pressure, and normal amounts of exercise in our lives. We should be able to walk and work and play and feel good. That's what's important.

Hypertension and Diabetes (Metabolic Syndrome)

June and Barbara: Since you've mentioned blood pressure, that gives us a chance to ask about another unpleasant statistic having to do with type 2 diabetes. To us it's astounding that between 45 and 50 percent of type 2s also have high blood pressure, and this is regardless of their ethnic background. How do you account for this, and what does it mean?

Virginia: It means that diabetes is more and more being recognized not as a single disease but as part of a group of diseases and possibly even the cause of all the diseases in the group. This larger problem is sometimes mysteriously called metabolic syndrome or, more descriptively, insulin resistance syndrome. I call it "hyperbetes," because its main features are hypertension and diabetes. Hypertension is the scientific word for high blood pressure.

I know this is a book about type 2 diabetes, but we must look at the bigger picture. Over half the people with type 2 either have or will get high blood pressure. The other diseases of metabolic syndrome are hyperlipidemia and atherosclerotic heart disease. Hyperlipidemia means high levels of fats in the blood, and in this case more is not better. Abnormal levels of blood lipids and high blood pressure over time lead to atherosclerotic heart disease (ASHD). This means that the blood vessels serving the heart are getting clogged up; when one or more of them become totally clogged, it causes a heart attack. People with type 2 diabetes die from heart disease more than from any other cause. When I am in the hospital to see patients, I end up spending more time on the heart floors than anywhere else, because over 30 percent of the patients there have diabetes. That is not a coincidence. This is why throughout this book we'll be talking about treating diabetes, but it may sound like we're treating heart disease instead. To determine if you may have metabolic syndrome, take the following test:

Measure (any three of five constitute diagnosis of metabolic syndrome)	Categorical Cutpoints
Elevated waist circumference	≥102 cm (≥40 inches) in men ≥88 cm (≥35 inches) in women
Elevated triglycerides	≥150 mg/dL (1.7 mmol/L) or On drug treatment for elevated triglycerides
Reduced HDL-C	<40 mg/dL (1.03 mmol/L) in men <50 mg/dL (1.3 mmol/L) in women or On drug treatment for reduced HDL-C
Elevated blood pressure	≥130 mm Hg systolic blood pressure or ≥85 mm Hg diastolic blood pressure or On antihypertensive drug treatment in a patient with a history of hypertension
Elevated fasting glucose	≥100 mg/dL or On drug treatment for elevated glucose

June and Barbara: We see there's a lot more to worry about than we realized and that we need to understand serious health problems other than diabetes. Why don't you take these terms—hypertension, hyperlipidemia, and atherosclerotic heart disease—and define each of them for us before we go on?

Virginia: Hypertension simply means high blood pressure. Normal blood pressure is about 120/80. Blood pressure over 130/80 is considered elevated. Hyperlipidemia means that you have high levels of lipids (fatty substances) in your blood. Blood lipids consist of triglycerides, cholesterol, and phospholipids. These circulate in your blood and are hooked up to proteins. That's why you may hear your doctor refer to them as lipoproteins. So now you may be asking, what are triglycerides and cholesterol?

TRIGLYCERIDES: These are the main storage forms of lipids and constitute about 95 percent of the fatty tissue of the body.

CHOLESTEROL: This is a natural component of cell membranes and is used to make other substances in the body, such as some hormones. Cholesterol can be absorbed from food or it can be manufactured by the liver. The kinds of cholesterol you hear about are HDL (high-density lipoprotein) and LDL (low-density lipoprotein). HDLs are known as "good lipids" because they are associated with decreased risk of heart disease. LDLs are known as "bad lipids" because a high level of LDLs has a strong and direct association with coronary artery disease. So you see, it is not enough to have a good total cholesterol anymore (under 200). You have to have high HDLs (above 50) and low LDLs (below 100). Now the National Cholesterol Education Program tells us that people with diabetes have even better survival from heart disease if they have an LDL less than 70. This usually requires a drug such as a statin. Statins are drugs such as Crestor, Lipitor, and Zocor. Zocor is now generic, called simvastatin, and another older generic statin is lo-vastatin. Statins have made a huge difference in the rate of heart disease in the United States in recent years but have some side effects for some people. The side effects can be muscle aches and pain. Some people can switch drugs and get rid of the aches, but for others the side effects persist and make taking a statin intolerable. Some patients tell me that taking coenzyme Q10 along with the statin prevents the aches. Another drug that boosts the effect of the statin is Zetia. By reducing the fat absorbed in the gut, your cholesterol is improved. You will see a combo med on the market that combines Zocor and Zetia, called Vytorin. Recently, some have found that Zetia did not change the amount of plaque in the blood vessels as much as statins even though the Zetia is effective for lowering LDL. Most of the endocrinologists I work with still use Zetia because the research studies on the positive side far outweigh the one small study that was negative. The study did not find that it caused harm.

Atherosclerotic heart disease is brought on by fat-clogged blood vessels that can cause a heart attack. The problems that contribute to ASHD are diabetes, high blood lipids, high blood pressure, and smoking. Smoking more than doubles your risk of ASHD, and it is something you can choose to do or not do. So don't do it.

June and Barbara: Besides not smoking, what can you do about hyperbetes?

Virginia: Hypertension and high blood lipids will improve if you follow our recommendation of a low-fat, low-salt diet and exercise. But remember that these problems are genetic, and if they don't get better with lifestyle changes, there are excellent medications that will help. Check with your doctor regarding your goal range for lipids and have them checked at least twice a year. Have your blood pressure checked at least every three months and have a goal of a systolic number (that's the top number) of less than 130 and a diastolic number (that's the bottom one) as close to 80 as possible. This is referred to as 130 over 80.

There are newer and better drugs for treating high blood pressure these days. They are classified as ACE (angiotensin converting enzyme) inhibitors. They have been found to be especially beneficial for people with diabetes in that they may have a protective effect on the kidneys. Check with your doctor about whether these drugs would be suited for you. Also, blood pressure medication is like diabetes medication in the sense that you may need it for a while and then, with weight loss and exercise, you may be able to discontinue it. That's why it's important to see your doctor and get your blood pressure checked every three months so that he or she can adjust your dose as needed.

June and Barbara: Are there any still newer and better drugs?

Virginia: About 5 percent of people on ACE inhibitor drugs will get a tickle cough that is very bothersome. For these people we can use the next level of angiotensin reduction, these are called ARBs, or angiotensin receptor blockers. Some people require both an ACE and an ARB to control their blood pressure. These drugs are particularly indicated when the patient is spilling microscopic protein in the urine (microalbuminuria), an indicator of kidney damage.

As you can see, hyperbetes is something we can all live with. One of our patients, Celia, is a good example. She came to us with all the classic symptoms. She had diabetes with an A1C of 10+ (see page 58 for a definition), she was about seventy pounds overweight, and she had high blood pressure and elevated lipids. She had the hypertension part of the syndrome before the diabetes; at least it was diagnosed first. She was put on a diuretic (water pill) for the high blood pressure, and it did what diuretics often do—it raised her blood sugar a little. This is one of the reasons that diuretics are not the best drug group to start with for high blood pressure control, although they may be needed later in people with diabetes.

Celia was sent to us for diabetes education, and we realized that the diuretic was probably the culprit. We suggested she consult one of our endocrinologists. Our docs put her on a better regimen of blood pressure–lowering medication plus oral agents for her diabetes. After a few months of working with our dietitians for diabetes control, she lost twenty-two pounds and was able to stop taking her blood pressure medication, her lipid-lowering drugs, and her diabetes pills. So you see, the diabetes lifestyle—low-fat diet, weight loss, exercise—works to treat the hyperbetes syndrome. Celia was thrilled, and we'll continue to work with her to help her stay in good control.

Don't get me wrong. There is nothing wrong with medications for treating blood pressure, lipids, and diabetes. We would all prefer to get along without them and as early in the disease as possible. But when it is not possible, it's important to follow the prescribed treatment.

WHITE COATS AND DARK CHOCOLATE

Before we leave the hypertension part of hyperbetes, I, Barbara, the member of the triumvirate without diabetes, have a little tale to tell. To my knowledge I've never had high blood pressure. At least no one of the medical persuasion ever told me I did. But then, during a routine exam, my doctor told me my blood pressure was "on the high side" and she seemed concerned about it. This really surprised me, so I checked myself on June's handy dandy Omron automatic blood pressure monitor. (As a conscientious person with diabetes, June has been daily taking her blood pressure for years.)

When I took my blood pressure at home it was perfectly normal, yet every time my doctor checked it, it was invariably "on the high side," and she started muttering about giving me a medication for it. Now, as Virginia said, it is important to treat hypertension to avoid heart disease and stroke, yet I've always tried not to take anything I don't really need.

I pondered the situation and decided that the problem must be that old devil white coat syndrome. It happens to many people, including several friends. As soon as they're in the vicinity of a health professional wearing the traditional white coat, up goes the blood pressure. My doctor didn't buy this diagnosis. In fact she doubted the accuracy of June's blood pressure monitor, not my veracity. She had me bring the monitor to the office so she could compare it with hers.

The good news is they lined up perfectly. The bad news was they both showed my blood pressure was on the high side. Well, why not?! After all, I was in the midst of a plethora of white coats.

So I decided I'd just relax and not worry—and hope my doctor did the same. Then two things happened:

1. I started occasionally having blood pressure readings that on June's meter were (you guessed it) on the high side. And gradually they became more frequent. How could this be? I wasn't doing anything different. My stress level was the same (rather high, as always). What was going on?

2. In doing research for this book, I began reading in the medical sections of newspapers that eating dark (*very* dark) chocolate could—in some cases—lower blood pressure. The author of one of the articles who tried the chocolate cure kind of shrugged it off, saying, in effect, that he really didn't have much confidence in it but since it did seem to keep his blood pressure lower, what harm could it do him? So he continued

with it. And what harm could it do to me? That, then, was my ultimate decision. I started eating one square of dark chocolate (Valrhona Le Noir Extra Amer—Dark Chocolate 85%) twice a day (occasionally three times).

My "on the high side" blood pressure at first stayed the same, then went down until it reached the point that I seldom if ever had a blood pressure over 130 unless I was in an extreme stress situation. **Note:** Today it was 114/68.

And so, for what it's worth, I offer you this blood pressure medication. It may be that a lot of it is in the head. Just as the white coat in the doctor's office unnerves me and raises my blood pressure, the dark chocolate soothes me and lowers it. Whatever.

While I'm at it, I have a couple more morsels of good news associated with this therapy:

1. Since it contains so much chocolate there's not much room for sugar, thereby eliminating a diabetes concern.
2. Stanley Marcus, the cofounder of the famed Neiman Marcus company, did not permit milk chocolate to be stocked in any of his stores. "Milk chocolate is a rube taste," he said. Hence, dark chocolate was the only kind of chocolate he'd allow to darken (!) their doors.

So there you have it. Dark chocolate *might* help lower your blood pressure, *should* do little or no harm to your diabetes, and definitely *would* enhance your reputation as a sophisticated person with refined taste. Who could ask for anything more?

Note: If this therapy doesn't work for you, remember what Virginia said: "There is nothing wrong with medications for treating blood pressure."

2

Ways and Means of Control

Doing What You Have to Do

NOW WE COME TO THE MAJOR UN-FUN PART OF DIABETES—the tedious, boring, relentless, day-after-day part. This is the testing of your blood sugar to see where you are and, in some cases, the taking of pills or insulin to get you where you want to be and keep you there.

Faced with this most unsatisfying aspect of diabetes, we need a little shot of philosophy. How about this one from Thomas Merton's *The Springs of Contemplation: A Retreat at the Abbey of Gethsemani*:

> If I insist that my work . . . mustn't be tedious or monotonous, I'm in trouble. . . . Time after time it fails to become so. So I get more agitated about it, I fight with people about it. I make more demands about it. It's ridicu-

lous to demand that work always be pleasurable, because work is not necessarily pleasing. . . . If we're detached and simply pick up the job we have to do and go ahead and do it, it's usually fairly satisfying. Even jobs that are repugnant and dull or tedious tend to be quite satisfying, once we get right down to doing them. This happens when we just do what we have to do.

That's the way it is with doing what we sometimes refer to as "diabetic shenanigans." June tests her blood sugar six or seven times a day and takes five separate injections—sometimes more if she's sick or changing time zones or her blood sugars have gone haywire for some other reason. If she got agitated and fought with people about having to do this, she'd be a one-woman war zone. No, she just does what she has to do.

It's not likely that you'll have this much tedium and travail in your life with diabetes, especially if you don't take insulin, but you still need to do what you have to do. And if you just do it without agitation, you'll find it's not so bad, maybe even quite satisfying, especially when you discover that you did what you had to do—and it worked.

There's another advantage to doing your diabetic shenanigans. It helps you keep your mind alert and your wits about you. Chief Justice Oliver Wendell Holmes Jr., who lived to be ninety-four, kept his mind sharp right up to the end by doing crossword puzzles every day. Being a person with diabetes means never having to look around for an activity to keep you on your mental toes. You've got one built in that will last your whole life.

—*June and Barbara*

Goals for Blood Sugar Levels

June and Barbara: What do health professionals mean when they say a person with diabetes is "in control" or "out of control"?

Virginia: This refers to how closely their blood glucose aligns with blood glucose goals. The general goals for diabetes control are 80 to 120 before meals, and 140 is the danger, or "take action," level. What finally led to more realistic goals for control was the 1993 release of the results of the Diabetes Control and Complications Trial (DCCT). This ten-year study followed 1,441 people with type 1 diabetes. It compared conventional treatment of two shots of insulin a day and one blood sugar test with intensive treatment of three or four shots of insulin a day and a minimum of four blood sugar tests a day. The DCCT proved that near normal blood glucose control can significantly help reduce the development of complications in type 1 patients.

Well, we all knew that metabolic control really matters, but we had no idea how positive the study would be. It was better than we ever dreamed. Diabetic retinopathy was reduced by 76 percent, kidney disease was prevented or delayed by 56 percent, and neuropathy (nerve damage) by 60 percent. I went to the American Diabetes Association meeting in Las Vegas and sat in the front row to hear the news. I just knew that patients would be beating my door down when I got back to work. The response was underwhelming. Most patients still don't know, and most doctors still don't believe the results. Many doctors claim it only applied to type 1 and didn't prove effective for type 2.

Then, the Kumamoto Study was published. This study replicated the DCCT on 110 type 2 patients in Japan. Guess what? The results came out pretty much the same as the DCCT for eye and kidney disease and even showed a 50 percent reduction in cardiac events. All the type 2s in the study were on insulin to manage their diabetes. Amazingly, there are still folks out there telling patients it's perfectly okay if their blood sugar is under 200. But now we know that good control makes a difference.

And to put the final piece in the puzzle of how low blood sugar can go for control, in the fall of 1998 the United Kingdom Prospective Diabetes Study announced the results of their twenty-year study of type 2 diabetes. This study of more than five thousand patients, enrolled as they were newly diagnosed, established that retinopathy, nephropathy, and neuropathy are benefitted by lowering glucose with intensive therapy. The intensive therapy achieved a median HbA1C of 7.0 percent compared to 7.9 percent in the conventional therapy group. This level of control decreased the overall complication rate by 25 percent. The study also found that cardiovascular complications were reduced by 16 percent but that these results were not "statistically significant." What that means is that it narrowly missed being a change that they could say with confidence would not have occurred by chance. They did find that for every 1 point decrease in HbA1C (such as 9 to 8 percent), there was a 25 percent reduction in diabetes-related deaths, a 7 percent reduction in mortality of all causes, and an 18 percent reduction in combined fatal and nonfatal myocardial infarction (heart attacks). They also found a positive benefit from lowering blood pressure to a mean of 144/82 in that it reduced strokes, heart failure, microvascular complications, and visual loss. I don't know about you, but these outcomes are enough evidence for me to want to get my glucose and blood pressure into really good control and keep it there.

June and Barbara: So what are your recommendations for each individual's goals for control now?

Virginia: "Individual" is the correct word because goals should be established individually for each person. For instance, a person who is nearly eighty years of age doesn't need goals that aim for intensive control. This kind of tight control is ideally designed to prevent complications down the road. When you're eighty, the complications that you fear thirty years from the time of diagnosis are pretty insignificant. You can settle for blood sugars in a range where you feel good. No matter what your age, you deserve to feel good.

Again, in an elderly person severe hypoglycemia (low blood sugar) should be avoided because it can be dangerous. It could lead to a serious fall, for example. Depending on the individual, we might extend the goal range to somewhat higher than the tighter control levels generally recommended for younger people. We keep in mind, though, that if blood sugars go too high, the elderly person will not feel good and will be at increased risk of dehydration and infections.

For most type 2s the American Association of Clinical Endocrinologists now recommends that glucose be maintained as near normal as possible. The organization suggests a fasting glucose less than 110 and after meals less than 140 at two hours and a AK of 6.5 or less. These may need to be modified for very young kids, elderly, or people with severe low glucose events. In those folks a fasting goal may be less than 140 and after meals less than 180. Those are near normal ranges—in other words, close enough to normal to prevent complications yet not so close to normal that we're constantly battling hypoglycemia (low blood sugar) if the person is on medication.

Some type 2s on insulin have severe hypoglycemic reactions with little or no warning. This sometimes happens to those who've had diabetes a long time because they lose their ability to sense the reactions. This is called hypoglycemic unawareness. Most people with diabetes can recognize an insulin reaction because of the typical symptoms of shaking, sweating, dizziness, poor coordination, and even less dramatic signs such as hunger, blurred vision, and irritability.

People who've developed hypoglycemic unawareness don't have these warning symptoms. They can get such a low blood sugar level that they suddenly pass out. This is why we tell them that it is their responsibility to test their blood sugar before they get behind the steering wheel of a car. Every time. And it should always be above 100 before they start out.

June and Barbara: June was subject to hypoglycemic unawareness for many years. Her blood sugar could drop to 40, and she wouldn't even know it. The solution to this problem is to work hard to normalize your blood sugar, and you will then regain awareness of your symptoms of lows. June switched to a low-carbohydrate diet in 1995 and was able to stay within a range of 70 to 100. After about two months, she totally regained her hypoglycemic warning symptoms and can now tell at a level of only 60. Let's switch now to another important problem:

Choosing a Doctor

When people are first diagnosed—and sometimes later on down the line—they ask, "How do I go about finding a physician who's really good at managing diabetes?"

Virginia: My advice would be to ask other people with diabetes and get their recommendations. If you don't know any other people with diabetes (not likely these days), you could call your local diabetes association and ask for the names of some doctors specializing in diabetes. If you don't have a local diabetes association, you could call a local hospital and ask which physicians on their staff specialize in diabetes. One thing to watch for when you're doctor-shopping is to find one who has a team of diabetes educators at his or her disposal. A doctor who does not use diabetes educator nurses and dietitians is not serious about managing diabetes.

June and Barbara: Most people already have a family doctor, and so their question is likely to be, "Is it okay to stay with my family doctor to take care of my diabetes or do I need to go to an expert, such as an endocrinologist or diabetologist?" Before you answer that, for the uninitiated, you'd better clarify exactly what these two specialists are and what they do.

Virginia: An endocrinologist is an internal medicine physician who has had additional training in endocrine diseases (those involving the secretion of various hormones). Usually he or she has had an additional two- or three-year fellowship and will probably be board certified in endocrinology. (**Tip:** Read the diplomas and certificates on the office wall.) Over half the patients of most endocrinologists have diabetes. It's by far the most common endocrine problem. Some endocrinologists refer to themselves as diabetologists because they specialize in the care of diabetes. A diabetologist can also be an internal medicine physician who did not take a fellowship in endocrinology but who specializes in diabetes in his practice.

June and Barbara: Now that we know what endocrinologists and diabetologists are, let's go back to the basic question: "Do I need one?"

Virginia: That's a question for each individual to decide. But there's help available in making your decision: the standards-of-care criteria written by the American Diabetes Association (ADA). These standards were developed by a consensus of top medical minds in diabetes and were designed to assure the best quality of care and also to be cost-effective. They are available from your local ADA affiliate. After reading them, you may ask yourself, "Am I getting this kind of monitoring of my progress and is my family physician capable of providing this level of monitoring?" If your answer is yes and you feel you have a good relationship with your doctor and are getting the continuity of care that is so important for a person with a chronic disease, then very likely you'll do fine with the doctor you have. It is also important, however, for you to have access to diabetes educators either through your doctor's office or elsewhere in the community.

On the other hand, an endocrinologist offers a different level of expertise in analyzing and treating the endocrine problems that you may be experiencing. You may need such help especially when you're just starting out your life as a person with diabetes. An initial consultation with an endocrinologist can put you on the right track for the best level of care and diabetes control.

Many people will decide to stay with the endocrinologist either because they have difficulty in achieving control or because their care is complicated by another problem, such as hypertension or a thyroid disorder, and they need the additional level of expertise of the endocrinologist in these areas.

Another time that an endocrinologist may be especially valuable is when you have had diabetes for many years and are starting to experience complications or are worried that you might develop them. In either case, you might need the services of an endocrinologist for complication screening and treatment.

June and Barbara: Is it an either/or situation? Once you decide to work with an endocrinologist, must you say farewell to your family doctor and the longtime relationship you've built up with him or her? ·

Virginia: Not at all. As I said before, you may feel you need an endocrinologist at the beginning, and then after you feel confident that your diabetes is in control and you can handle it, you can go back to your family doctor.

Then, too, you can be under the care of a primary-care physician and use an endocrinologist as a consultant who only works with you on your diabetes problems. Your family doctor is the one who takes care of your everyday sniffles and sore throats and flus and your other general medical problems. This is the best solution for many people.

June and Barbara: Is the best solution always possible? Doesn't your health insurance provider or your HMO tell you what you have to do when it comes to seeking help for your diabetes?

Virginia: That's true. Many times the third-party payment systems require that you go to your primary-care physician for basic care, and they only let you see an endocrinologist if your primary care physician thinks it's necessary and gives you a referral to one.

June and Barbara: What happens when you think you need to consult an endocrinologist and your primary-care physician thinks you don't?

Virginia: Although that sounds like an impossible tug-of-war for you, there is someone available to put some weight on your end of the rope. Health maintenance organizations have care managers or benefit supervisors to help resolve such situations. They may negotiate with your primary-care physician to give you at least an initial referral, or they may even assign you to a different primary-care physician. This latter might be the better idea, since if the disagreement has gone this far, it may have undermined the doctor-patient relationship to the point that you can no longer work effectively together.

Let me emphasize something here: it doesn't pay to be shy when it comes to your personal health-care needs. Nobody is giving nice-guy points when it comes to taking care of your own health needs. You must realize, too, that no one—health professional or not—will take the level of responsibility for your health care that you yourself will. It is especially important for you to develop this attitude of self-responsibility in this day and age when all the health-care systems are looking for the most cost-effective ways to deliver health care. You have to be strong, capable, and well-informed if you want to have the care you need and deserve.

June and Barbara: That reminds us of our friend Jean, a college professor. She was in the hospital several days for extensive tests. Whenever she felt the care she received was inept or ineffective, she let the hospital staff know about it in no uncertain terms and demanded that the situation be rectified immediately. She almost always got what she wanted. As she was leaving the hospital, and had mellowed out somewhat because of the favorable results of her stay, she remarked to a nurse, "I guess I'm known around here as the scourge of the fifth floor."

"No," replied the nurse, smiling sweetly, "the scourge of the whole west wing."

Now, being obnoxious in general just because you're unhappy at being sick or incapacitated doesn't help matters in health care any more than it does in any other area of life. But we agree with Virginia (and know from our own experience) that a little scourging at the right time can work wonders when you are being denied the care—or the endocrinologist—that you know you need.

But we should mention here that an endocrinologist isn't the only key to your diabetes success. In fact one isn't always necessary, as is pointed out in this well-reasoned response to "Beating the Goalie," an article published in the *Diabetic Reader* explaining how to get through an HMO "gatekeeper" to a specialist.

> While I appreciate the frustration that your readers may feel about the HMO system, I would disagree that all people with diabetes need to see a specialist for regular medical care. While it is important to see a practitioner who follows ADA guidelines and is up-to-date on diabetes care, it does not necessarily follow that this physician needs to be a specialist.
>
> As a family practitioner providing care to a large number of people with diabetes, I try to assure that all of my patients receive recommended lab work, follow up frequently with a diabetes educator, check their blood sugars at home, and are screened regularly for early signs of complications. Because I am a family practitioner, I also make sure they receive regular Pap smears, mammograms, screening for colon cancer and prostate cancer, and other routine health care. I do have some patients whose diabetes is too complicated for me and I readily refer the patient to an endocrinologist. I also refer anyone who feels they need a consultation to a specialist.
>
> More important than the type of specialist is the doctor herself. Finding a doctor who keeps herself well educated, knows her limitations, and whom you feel you can trust is essential. If you find this doctor, then regardless of whether this person is a family practitioner, internist, or

specialist, I would urge you to do anything you can to convince your HMO that she is the one you need to see.

This letter is right on. Actually, June has a doctor she feels she can trust and he happens to be a gynecologist. She particularly likes him because he lets her be the captain of her diabetes therapy ship, and whenever she wants to try something new or unorthodox, he guides and supports her. As June says jokingly, "I love a compliant doctor." Before we leave the realm of the endocrinologist, is there any time in life when a person with diabetes definitely requires the services of one?

Virginia: Absolutely. During pregnancy. Any woman with diabetes who is even thinking about having a baby should be under the care of an endocrinologist. In the first place, you want to be in good diabetes control before getting pregnant, since most of the damage the baby might receive from a mother with out-of-control diabetes takes place in the first trimester. Then, after you become pregnant, you'll probably also want to work with a perinatologist, a physician who specializes in high-risk obstetrics. If you can find a diabetes pregnancy team, this is the most effective way to manage the problems of diabetes and pregnancy. The dream team would consist of the following:

- Endocrinologist
- Perinatologist
- Obstetrician
- Diabetes nurse educator
- Diabetes dietitian educator
- Genetic counselor
- Social worker

Call your local diabetes association to find such a diabetes and pregnancy program. It's certainly more complicated for a woman with diabetes to have a baby, but with the proper care and attention on her part and on the part of the health professionals she works with, she can have a healthy, happy baby just like any other woman.

June and Barbara: Do you have any other tips for being an effective diabetes manager?

Virginia: Yes, I would recommend to anyone, whether they have diabetes or not, that they keep their own medical records. There is very little about the health-care system that is computerized. It is still largely a paper-based system, subject to loss and misplacement. We have learned that it is best if you keep your own central chart, particularly if you are changing physicians or going from specialist to specialist. Every time you see your doctor and see he is looking at a lab report, ask for a copy. When a specialist says, "I will send a report to your primary-care physician," pipe up and say, "Please send a copy to me as well." If you have a physician who does not want to share that information with you, you may be spending your money on the wrong doctor. You must insist that every procedure, every lab report, and even your physician's notes be copied to you, and keep them in a notebook. Write up your own brief history of medical conditions and list allergies, medications, and treatments; take a copy every time you see your doctor. This way they don't have to thumb through your chart to find this information. I know my doctor really appreciates this information. I keep it in a file on my computer, and then we have no confusion about what the doctor thinks I am taking and what I am really taking.

Glycohemoglobin Test

June and Barbara: Lots of doctors don't seem all that interested in their patients' daily blood sugar tests. They act as if the only really important thing is the glycohemoglobin (HbA1C) test. Maybe you should explain what this laboratory test is and why doctors consider it so important.

Virginia: A lot is changing in this important monitoring test. A few years ago, the ADA and all the other big organizations decided that we had too many names for the same test and patients are confused. They decided to call it the A1C test. This is helping a little, but I still have patients ask for their A1C test result. Now the large organizations are planning to change again. They are looking into new technology that makes long-term control monitoring more accurate with fewer interfering substances and also changing the way we report the results. They are considering going to "average blood glucose" as the measure so that people don't have to convert a number that doesn't mean anything to them into an average glucose to be able to relate it to control. We will see how this progresses over the next few years.

I've known physicians who consider the A1C to be the most important—if not the only important—test for their patients. To put it simply, this test analyzes how much glucose has bonded with your red blood cells and, thereby, indicates what your average blood sugars have been for the past eight to ten weeks (the time varies from individual to individual). It's a test that must be attended to since it most closely aligns with risks for the complications of diabetes. This makes it an extremely important indicator; a kind of shining beacon to the person with diabetes to illuminate what the future may hold. Certainly we all want to pay attention to the results of this test, to understand what it means, and, above all, to strive to stay within our goal range, which is 1/2 to 1 point above the top of the normal range (usually this means your goal is 6.5 or 7 or less). The ADA recently stated that in selected individuals, the goal may be an A1C of 6 or less. Certainly, if you can achieve an A1C in the normal range, you should go for it. I think Mother Nature had a plan and I am always happy to go along with "normal." I can really tell the difference between an A1C of 7 and one that is less than 6. At 7 you feel good, but below 6 you start to realize that you feel normal, which is about 10 times better than good. I am now able to maintain an A1C of 4.9 to 5 percent and feel great.

You may notice that next time your doctor does an A1C test in the office from a finger stick, you will get results in five or six minutes. These tests are quite accurate and really improve the value of the visit because your doctor can discuss the results and make changes immediately. If the A1C test is so important, why bother doing daily blood sugars? Because you can't fix a poor A1C result unless you know what your daily blood glucose levels are—day in and day out—and work to improve those.

To sum up: The A1C test is your long-term beacon. Your blood glucose tests tell you how you're doing in controlling your diabetes on a day-to-day basis. The daily tests give you the clues as to where your control problems are and what you need to do to improve. These two tests go hand in hand like love and marriage. Both are absolutely necessary if you want really good control.

Urine and Blood Glucose Testing

June and Barbara: Some people with diabetes are first told to test the amount of sugar in their urine to help with their control (this is the old-fashioned way), while others are put directly onto blood glucose testing. What is the difference between testing urine and blood?

Virginia: It's very simple: urine testing is worthless and blood testing is not. To go into a little more detail, urine glucose measurements are, as you put it, the old-fashioned way. Many years ago, when there was no technology available for blood sugar testing at home, urine sugar measurements were thought to give some reflection of blood glucose variations that could be used to keep people in control. Since you don't "spill" (another old-fashioned term) glucose into your urine until your blood sugar is higher than about 180 to 200 (and even higher than that if you're older), then urine testing isn't going to be of much value. Added to that problem is the fact that urine glucose testing varies with the amount of liquid in the bladder. You may have had a spike of high sugar and then low sugar and you'll still spill glucose into your urine, even though at the time of testing your blood sugar is very low.

Let me give you an analogy. Testing urine for glucose control of diabetes is like driving a car using only the rearview mirror. As far as I'm concerned, it has no value. Some people say, "Yes, but it costs less money." Not really. When you consider the value of the information you get, it's extremely expensive. People also say that it's better than nothing. Au contraire. I'd like to assert that it's worse than nothing. Too often you're getting a false sense of security. Many people with type 2 diabetes don't spill glucose into their urine until their blood sugars are in the 300 range (usually older people). As long as they're getting negative urine tests, they think they're doing okay, when in fact they're not.

Did I say urine test strips were worthless? Actually, they do have one useful function. They're great for testing diet soft drinks. Did you know that from 10 percent to 26 percent of fountain "diet" soft drinks may be regular soda instead? One of the teens we take care of did this test at a mall in Albuquerque. He used urine testing strips to test Diet Coke ordered at all the places where it was available in the mall. More than 10 percent were the real thing and not diet. At one food outlet an employee confessed, "We were out of Diet Coke so we hooked up real Coke." Our patient explained to the employee that this deceptive practice could seriously hurt a person with diabetes. You can be sure the employee won't do that again.

June and Barbara: We've had lots of people report this nondiet diet-drink phenomenon to us. Some who have checked it out have found even higher percentages of "mistakes," up to one-third the wrong thing. You can also use urine test strips to check salad dressings and sauces. If they register below 1/2 percent glucose on Diastix or a urine glucose strip, they're probably safe. Let's move on now to the subject of blood glucose testing, which is far from worthless.

Virginia: Glucose monitors have become very accurate, small, and fast. Most now take an extremely small amount of blood and give an accurate result in less than six seconds. They keep track of results and some even allow you to tag the result as being before or after a meal. I know of one monitor that will be coming on the market in the next year that draws up the blood with the lance and deposits the sample on the reagent in one swift move in less than five seconds. Now most of the best monitors also code themselves; in other words, you don't have to enter a code number or chip to calibrate the system to each batch of strips. But all these labor-saving features still don't take into account the most important step; that is, stopping what you are doing and turning your focus to doing the test. Even though the test only takes a few seconds and the lancing devices are virtually pain-free, they don't do the test for you. The biggest problem we have with blood glucose monitoring is that patients don't do it, or don't do it often enough and at the right time.

June and Barbara: Assuming cost is a prime consideration, at what time of day should people take their blood sugar tests and exactly how often? Different doctors suggest different schedules. Tell us what plan you recommend and why.

Virginia: That depends on what information you need to know. Let me go through the different testing times and what they're telling you. First of all, most of you need to test your fasting (before breakfast) blood glucose to find out how you're starting the day. This tells us how you're managing your blood glucose without the impact of food. Since most type 2s have high fasting levels (remember that excess liver metabolism phenomenon), even though they may be better off the rest of the day, it's important to know that as well.

Now let's talk about testing after meals. If you really want to know how food is affecting your blood glucose, test one or two hours after the meal. This is a true look at how the carbohydrate is affecting your blood glucose. For people using diet alone to manage their blood glucose, this is important information. Don't expect your postmeal blood glucose to be the same as your fasting blood glucose. Notice that when I gave you your goals for control there were two different sets, one for fasting and one for after meals.

If you're on medication, that's a different story. Many times your doctor has instructed you to test before meals. This is the number you need to know to determine how well the medication is working. For instance, your fasting blood glucose tells you how well the oral diabetes medication you took at supper is working or how well the long-acting insulin that you took last night is working. Many times if you get your fasting blood glucose in the normal range, then the rest of the day works out a lot better. Your before-lunch blood sugar is reflective of both the short-acting insulin that covered breakfast, as well as the long-acting insulin you take to cover the whole day. Sometimes you also have to look at your before-supper blood sugar to get an idea of how you might adjust your morning insulin. It also tells you how well the pill or long-acting insulin you took in the morning is working.

To sum it up for people on medication, probably a before-breakfast and a before-supper test plus an occasional after-meal test would be an adequate schedule. One of the after-meal tests could be done at bedtime. That gives you an idea of how supper is affecting your blood glucose and how well your blood glucose is in control before you go to sleep. If you take long-acting insulin and are very low before bedtime, you need to plan for a snack.

If you're the kind of person who does a lot of strenuous exercise (I hope you are), you should be testing right before your workout. If your blood glucose is below 150, have a snack before you begin your exercise. (The 150 may be a somewhat high or low number for you; it can vary with individuals and the intensity of the exercise.) For those of you on medication, this test is a useful tool to keep you at your best blood sugar level for exercise. Exercise lowers blood sugar. Many people also test after their workout.

You should definitely test if you're feeling the symptoms of low blood sugar (sweating, shakiness, nervousness, weakness, confusion). You need to see at what level your blood sugar causes you to have these symptoms of hypoglycemia. Some people get symptoms at 120, while others might not feel low even at 40. Anytime you feel hypoglycemic, test to see how low you are and if you really need to eat something.

June and Barbara: There must be more than twenty models of blood sugar–testing meters available now from different manufacturers, and new ones seem to be coming on the market every other day. They're all different prices and have many different features. Let's say you're a newly diagnosed diabetes patient, and your health insurance will reimburse you for a meter and the monthly supply of strips to use with it, or that you can afford to pay the expenses yourself. How do you go about acquiring a meter you'll be happy with and trust?

Virginia: Let me give you a few criteria you can use:

1. Buy a meter made by a company you can trust. It doesn't necessarily have to be one of the major manufacturers that has been in business a long time. It could be a young company that's doing a good job of providing a meter system and support. But I'm always a little leery of a brand-new company with a brand-new meter. I can't tell you how many meters have come on the market for a short time, and then disappeared. Some models are shown at conventions for diabetes educators and then never even make it to market. Many of my patients have been stuck with a meter from a company that doesn't support it. By support I mean the company has a toll-free phone number answered by knowledgeable, pleasant, patient customer-service representatives who are empowered to replace your machine quickly if you're having any problems. Also, they should provide easy-to-understand literature and instructions with the machine.

2. Talk to your diabetes educator before you go to the drugstore to buy a monitor. You will be surprised to find out that your educator has a whole closet full of free meters and you should

probably not ever buy a monitor. Some of the TV advertise-ments for free meters and strips will give you a no-name meter that is questionable for accuracy and the mail-order business will bill full price to Medicare.

3. Go for a system that supports you in your lifestyle. If you're on the move a lot, go for a model that's small and easy to carry around, easy to use, easily understood, and that's accurate. If having a meter in your pocket or purse means you're more likely to do testing, then by all means, get an easily portable machine.

By and large, pharmacists are not experts on meter systems, al-though some have taken the time and effort to learn about meters. For the most part, pharmacists are experts on drugs and medica-tions; they're not experts on the stuff in front of the counter. So I suggest you talk to a diabetes educator. The educator has training and experience with meters, has spent time out there with people who are actually using meters, and probably knows more about these systems than any other health professional, including your doctor.

June and Barbara: Getting all those drops of blood to put on strips is no fun, as you well know. Many people—especially older people—have difficulty. Back when Barbara was teaching the use of meters and found someone who bled easily, she would go into raptures over them. ("You just bleed wonderfully! How lucky you are. If only everyone could get blood for their tests as easily as you do, this world would be a better place.") After you get the drop, put-ting it on the strip correctly can be an even greater ordeal. And when you botch the job, not only have you wasted an expensive strip, but you have to start all over again with a new drop. Do you have any magic solutions for avoiding all the above bloody mishaps?

Virginia: I don't know if they're magic, but there certainly are solutions. If you're one of those people who don't bleed easily, you should wash your hands in warm water before taking the test. Next, hold your hand down at your side below your hips. If you're sitting in a chair, let your hand hang straight down for a few minutes. This will allow it to fill up with blood.

Some people who have a particularly hard time getting blood find they have to really milk the finger. In this case, it helps if you practice doing this motion the right way. Starting way down at the base of the finger near your hand, milk all the way down the length of the finger to the tip on the palm side of the finger until you get a big drop. Then let go of the finger. Let your finger pink up again, then repeat the milking motion. Some people make the mistake of constantly squeezing the finger, never letting go to allow the blood to come back into the finger.

You should always stick your finger on the sides instead of on the fingerprint surface. The "poochy" sides of your finger actually bleed better. Another thing I suggest is to always stick the underneath side of your finger as opposed to the top side. That way the blood goes onto the strip easily and correctly. If you stick the top side of your finger, the blood tends to drip into your fingernails. This not only makes it hard to get the right amount of blood on the strip, but it's unsightly to walk around with blood under your nails.

The typical textbook on diabetes tells you not to stick in the same place all the time because you will get a callus. Most experienced people with diabetes know that a callus can be rather welcome because finger pricks in a callus don't hurt. When you get a callus so thick that you can no longer get blood, then you need to move on to other areas.

June and Barbara: The well-known diabetologist with diabetes Peter Forsham also suggested using this callus technique for people who're afraid of damaging their fingers with numerous finger sticks, such as musicians. He advised a concert pianist to take the finger he used least in his playing and always take the test from the same place on that finger, causing a callus to develop there.

June figures that she takes more than two thousand blood sugars a year, but the punctures haven't ruined her fingers in any way. Is this an unusual experience? Do some people with diabetes have problems with soreness and damaged fingers?

Virginia: Unfortunately, some people's fingers get so sore that they can hardly bear the thought of taking another blood sugar test. That's why I personally like to stick only the three fingers that have developed calluses thick enough to prevent pain.

But it's also very important to find the right lancing device. Some stick too deep for a particular individual. On the other hand, some don't stick deep enough to get the amount of blood needed for the test. The latest improvement in lancing devices is a feature that lets you "dial up" the depth of the stick. Your lancing device can be dialed down for tender thin skin or up to a depth sufficient for lizard-skinned fingers. Visit your diabetes educator, who usually has a whole drawer full of lancets. You can try out several to find the right one.

June and Barbara: June likes the auto-Lancet, which has a tip that adjusts with five settings to match your skin type. She's also found that the lancet can make a difference. Certain brands may stick deeper or shallower, and some are more painful than others.

Virginia: That's certainly true. My favorite lancet of the moment is the Accu-Chek Softclix. It does use the Softclix lancets, which are very fine and don't leave a big hole in my finger, although they don't fit most of the other lancing devices. I personally don't like having different lancets for different lancers because patients get confused about what to buy and pharmacies are generally of no help with this kind of trivia. Actually, I use the lancets over and over, so a box lasts me a long time.

June and Barbara: What if you think the meter you're using just gave you a wrong result—a totally unexpected and inexplicable number? This phenomenon usually only happens with an excessively high result. For some reason, we all are usually quite willing to accept readings on the low side as valid. In the case of the "wrong" reading, the normal reaction is to start cursing the meter. Some people may even want to hurl the thing across the room. They may actually do it. What do you suggest doing in such cases?

Virginia: This has certainly happened to all of us. Rather than cursing the meter and throwing it across the room, the first thing you would want to consider is whether this truly could be a meter error. As far as I'm aware, there hasn't been a meter made that won't give you an erroneous number at some point in its life. To check this out, you should retest, but first do some troubleshooting.

Wash your hands and retest, because traces of food—especially fruit—on your hands can be read by the meter and give you a false high reading.

Check the meter to see if it's clean. Do a control test using a drop of control solution that comes with your meter to see if the machine comes up with a number that falls within the acceptable range for the solution. The control test is good for checking both the meter and the strips. The problem is that it costs you a strip to do it.

Consider whether the temperature of the meter may be too hot or too cold, because that will affect how it is working. If, for example, the meter has been left in the car and is very warm or very cold to the touch, let it come back to room temperature before you proceed. Then retest your blood, being careful that your technique is exactly right and that you're putting the right amount of blood on the strip and doing the timing correctly. This is why I prefer systems that require very little technique. It's much easier not to make mistakes.

At this point, if the reading you get is drastically different from the first one, you have to ask yourself which reading was accurate. If, however, both of your meter readings agree fairly closely—as usually happens—then you have to admit to yourself that your blood sugar is indeed in that range, surprising though it may be.

June and Barbara: Let's talk about strips and meters and how the costs of both have changed. Back in the olden days when June first started testing her blood sugar, meters were expensive. Her first one, an Ames Eyetone Reflectance Meter, cost $350 used. Had she bought a new one, it would have been $650. On the other hand, at that time, strips were relatively inexpensive—45 to 50 cents apiece.

Then the meter manufacturers got onto the razor blade theory. That's the marketing idea Gillette discovered long ago. The razor is sold for very little because the manufacturer knows it then has a longtime customer for its blades, and the blade prices can be on the high side. As a result, meter prices have dropped to as low as free.

Where is the best place to buy a meter?

Virginia: I have found that if you're learning to monitor your blood sugar for the first time, you should purchase supplies from someone who can provide individualized education on blood sugar testing in general and on the meter you're purchasing in particular. Some medical supply stores can do this, although sometimes you're getting your instruction from a clerk with no specialized training in patient education or monitors.

A diabetes educator will probably be your best resource for training, and many times the educator will provide you with a meter or direct you to the best place to get one. Then you can bring the meter in for your training during a visit with the diabetes educator.

It's true that the meter may be the least expensive at a mail-order or discount pharmacy. If, however, because of lack of instruction, you do the test wrong and waste strips and get false readings that lead you to taking the wrong amount of medication, the savings wouldn't be worth it.

We've decided at the Diabetes Network that our main business is not selling meters, so we don't. We always suggest the discount or mail-order sources to our experienced patients who are upgrading to a newer model or who are buying a spare meter. You shouldn't have to pay for training if you don't need it. Still, it's a good idea to talk to your educator before you order some sensational deal from a catalog. We may be able to tell you why the meter is so cheap (for instance, it may be a meter that they're closing out because a newer and much better model will soon be available) or warn you of potential problems (such as you can only get the strips in Outer Mongolia on the fifth Tuesday of the month).

Another big plus for learning from a diabetes educator is that we are often the ones to find out about new stuff first. Recently, I got my hands on the new Medtronic implantable sensor. This marks a whole new leap in technology for glucose monitoring. Right now, the sensor reads glucose for three days; the information is then downloaded into a computer, so it is primarily for diagnostic or data collection purposes. They now also have an implantable sensor that transmits to a receiver in the insulin pump so that you can get continuous glucose readings and trends right on the pump screen. The DexCom system now has a seven-day sensor that reads glucose for a one-week period before it has to be changed. Abbott's FreeStyle Navigator system reads for five days and will soon transmit to pumps so that the patient does not have to wear two "boxes." Continuous glucose monitoring is certainly the future for monitoring, and it accounts for that important first step I alluded to earlier—that is, it does the test every few minutes without action on the part of the person with diabetes. Downside? Well, they aren't as accurate point to point as the monitors, but they tell you the trend of that reading. In other words, is that 110 on its way up or down or staying the same? And the biggest problem, they are very expensive. They can cost from $800 to $1,000 initially and then between $300 and $500 a month for the disposable supplies. There is also a fair amount of hassle factor in wearing something continuously on your body with the receiver hanging on you or nearby. I think the future will see these systems refined and improved and, hopefully, cheaper. Right now, few insurance companies are covering the cost of these systems.

June and Barbara: One thing we've noticed is that people often don't want to pay for diabetes education. They're willing to buy equipment and supplies because those are things they can hold in their hands and carry out the door. But in reality, the most valuable commodity they can buy is a better understanding of diabetes care. There's a Chinese proverb that we particularly like: "Put your money in your head, and nobody can take it away from you."

Part of the problem may be that insurance companies are sometimes reluctant to pay for education. This is a penny-wise and pound-foolish approach, since well-educated diabetes patients are more likely to stay out of the hospital where they'll run up huge bills for the insurance company to cover.

Virginia: I couldn't agree more! Many studies have shown clearly that patient education pays off in reduced hospitalizations and better health outcomes for the person with diabetes. The news about reimbursement and insurance coverage for diabetes education and supplies is now mostly positive. In the last few years, twenty-nine states have passed legislation mandating that health insurance companies pay for diabetes education and supplies. (New Mexico passed a bill several years ago.) In general, these statutes require coverage for diabetes education, meters, strips, and medications without regard to the type of diabetes or treatment.

Of course, states cannot make Medicare do anything, but Newt Gingrich and Bill Clinton actually agreed on something a few years ago and signed into law changes that will make Medicare pay for strips and meters for everybody, regardless of the type of diabetes or treatment. Medicare limits the number of strips to about one a day for people not on insulin and three a day for people on insulin. I have been successful getting some of my patients extra strips with a lot of paperwork and groveling. Medicare is getting ready to make a big change that might affect all of us. Starting this year in a limited number of cities, it will go into a "competitive bidding" mode where it will limit the number of suppliers and meter selection. This will spread over the next few years to cover most of the country. Most of us diabetes educators feel that this is not a good move. Medicare is doing it, of course, to save money. It sees meters and strips as a commodity like bedpans and wheel-chairs. We see that there are many types of monitors with specific features that fit different patient needs. I fear that the next step will be to limit even further the number of strips available.

I can see Medicare's point. According to data, only about half the patients with type 2 diabetes do glucose monitoring and they only test three to four times a week. I find that patients who don't test are the ones who have never been to a diabetes educator. Glu-cose monitoring is probably the most important activity that a person with diabetes can perform. It is the "biofeedback" that is so important, learning how medications, food, and activity are af-fecting your glucose so you can make changes appropriately.

And then, keeping track! Most of the meters have extensive memories but they don't remember what you had for lunch or what you were doing to cause your glucose to go low or high. That's why I encourage people to keep a log book for at least three weeks before our appointment so we can see what's affecting their glucose results. I am often disappointed because so many people come to their appointment with no meter or log book. My friend Debbie Hinnen reminds her patients: "Going to see your educator without your meter is like going to the vet without the dog."

Medicare covers diabetes education provided by certified dia-betes educators in Recognized Diabetes Education Programs. The ADA recognizes diabetes education programs which have com-pleted a rigorous quality process that requires a great amount of time and paper every three years with annual updates. The payment is meager and almost not worth sending a bill. I guess I shouldn't be ungrateful, but, sadly, many educators try to manage a business based on Medicare reimbursement and find that they can't make a living. We see Medicare patients in our group under the education benefit, but we find it is a deal for us and the patient to bill as providers—that is, because three of us in our practice are clinical nurse specialists (like a nurse practitioner, only we just do diabetes).

There is good news and bad news in Medicare paying for diabetes education. When Medicare starts paying for something and then sets a fee structure, it tends to set the standard that all other payers follow. My feeling is that most of the large insurance companies recognize the value of diabetes education in helping patients improve control, and they definitely appreciate the value of improved control. They needed education to be mandated so that it "levels the playing field." This means that all companies have to pay for the benefit and therefore the smaller companies don't have an advantage with paying fewer benefits and charging a lower premium. Speaking of the value to insurance companies, in Decem-

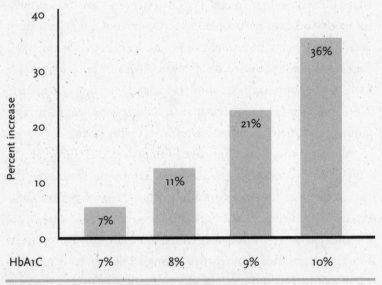

Figure 2.1 • Cost to health plans of poor glycemic control

Increase in medical charges over a three-year period for adults with diabetes and various HbA1C values of 6 percent. Adapted from Gilmer, T. P., et al. "The cost to health plans of poor glycemic control." Diabetes Care 20(12): 1847 (1997).

ber 1997, *Diabetes Care* published an article that demonstrated the impact of control on cost to health plans. This exciting information showed the increase in costs to the health plan of various A1C levels in patients who tested over 6 percent (see Figure 2.1). This is an excellent resource to use when you're trying to get an insurance company to pay for something to help you get into better control—it shows the value of control to the payer!

Keeping Records

June and Barbara: Is keeping records of your blood sugar tests absolutely essential? Recording the results is a lot of trouble, and what good is it—especially if you keep getting more or less the same numbers and they're all too high? We've had people show us their records and have been amazed that day in and day out they'll write down the same 240s, 280s, or 310s and not question the pointlessness of keeping track of the same bad blood sugars without getting the message that something different has to be done. Surely blood sugar testing isn't an end in itself.

Virginia: I agree that keeping records of blood sugars without taking any action is pointless. But I really encourage patients to keep track of their blood sugars while they are coming in for consultations with the diabetes educators. These records can help them identify areas of behavior that are causing them problems. For instance, we can correlate the high blood sugars with changes in diet, medication, or exercise. Also, by identifying patterns in the blood sugar readings we can help them change their medication to correct the problems.

But most important, while we're reviewing the records of their food intake, blood sugars, and exercise, we can help them learn our decision-making process. This is most important. Fine-tuning diabetes control is not rocket science. It's just being very sensitive to a person's lifestyle. We're never judgmental about blood sugars, and we teach the patients not to be judgmental, either. Blood sugars don't have anything to do with a person's character. They simply represent the effects of medication, exercise, food, and lifestyle on that particular individual. With time and practice you can learn how to make the adjustments in these factors just as well as a health professional can. And you will often have a choice in how to make these adjustments. For example, some people may choose to take more insulin or alter their medication to cover a particular meal or period of stress. Others may choose to exercise more. A lot of variations are possible. There isn't an absolute, rigid, you-must-live-this-way diabetes control program for everybody. We feel these choices should be left up to you, the patient. But you can't make these choices intelligently unless you're taught how. And you can be taught. Certainly if physicians can learn it and I can learn it and the health-care team I work with can learn it, you can learn it, too.

We've learned it because we practice, but mostly we've learned it because our patients have taught us. We take our patients' records and examine them and have the patients tell us what happened. Then, when we've done this often enough, we come up with some guidelines.

For example, we may say, "Gee, it looks like every time somebody has had pan pizza, their blood sugars are much higher than when they eat thin-crust pizza. There must be a pattern here." You can do this kind of analysis on yourself. You can also see, using your blood sugar tests, the different effects of exercise and medication. It's really not a terribly difficult decision-making process. The important part of it is learning to be creative and flexible and to realize that there's more than one way to skin a cat.

Medication: Pills and Insulin and Lizard Spit!

June and Barbara: You mentioned in your introduction that you managed your diabetes with diet for the first eight years of the disease and then went on to pills and eventually insulin. Now you're on some new therapies. What are these medications?

Virginia: True, when I was diagnosed I was on insulin for the first eight or nine months and lost about fifty pounds. With that amount of weight loss I was able to get off insulin and maintain good control with diet and exercise. Over the years, I have been on everything. Let's start with talking about the oldest of the diabetes oral medications. These medications are specifically for the treatment of type 2 diabetes. Now there are lots of new options compared to when I was diagnosed. We used to have only the sulfonylureas, which have been used for forty years. (This is pronounced sul-faw-nuhl-u-ree-us. It took me two years to learn how to say this. That's why most of us just call them pills.) Today we have several choices, and most are generic. These pills kick your pancreas to make a little more insulin. Some people think these medications will "wear out" your pancreas quicker, but this is controversial. The United Kingdom Prospective Diabetes Study (UKPDS) found that neither sulfonulureas nor metformin have that effect on insulin production. Interestingly, the study showed that whether a patient was on diet and exercise, sulfonylureas, metformin, or insulin, "pancreatic poop-out" was progressive and eventually people made less and less insulin and control deteriorated. Later, you will find out that we now may have the answer to stop this deterioration.

Among the new drugs that have appeared since 1995 are Glucophage (metformin), a group of drugs called TZDs (thiazolidinediones), and Precose (acarbose). Let me tell you about these and how they work and their drawbacks.

GLUCOPHAGE (METFORMIN): This is a recent cousin of a thirty-year-old drug. It can have some nasty side effects, but the trick is not to use it on people who are likely to get lactic acidosis (a side effect where the body doesn't eliminate wastes), as it can be fatal; some deaths have been reported from metformin (trade name Glucophage). People who have kidney damage are also not candidates for this drug. Before considering the drug, you should have a creatinine level drawn. Creatinine clearance is a measure of kidney function because this is a substance that clears from the body through the kidneys, and, if it is high, it means the kidneys aren't working to "clear" this substance as efficiently as they should. When you get a basic "metabolic panel" lab test, this will be one of the tests included. If it is above normal, your doctor may want to consider not using metformin. Another group of people at risk are those with poor liver function (people whose lab tests show abnormal liver function) and people who are binge drinkers or who drink significant amounts of alcohol. Additionally, people with congestive heart failure, COPD (chronic obstructive pulmonary disease), or any other serious disease should not be using metformin.

Now the good news. Metformin works by suppressing the liver's production of glucose. It does so by a totally different mechanism than the sulfonylureas, and can be combined with them to work together. As it turns out, either sulfonylurea or metformin will lower your fasting blood glucose about 50 to 60 mg/dl, but together they work better than either one alone. Some physicians still start with one of the sulfonylureas as the first-line therapy, but now many are starting with metformin and then adding the sulfonylurea for the second line. The American Diabetes Association and the American Association of Clinical Endocrinologists are now recommending metformin as the initial medication, and many recommend it even when a person has prediabetes or impaired glucose tolerance, since it was shown in the Diabetes Prevention Study to reduce progression to diabetes by 30 percent. When starting metformin, it is important to begin with one or two tablets a day (500 mg) with a meal for a week or so, and then add another tablet with another meal. For example, start with one 500 mg tablet with breakfast and supper; after one week add another 500 mg tablet at supper. Most people need to get their dose up to 1,500 to see the effect. The maximum dosage is 2,500, but studies have shown that 2,000 is as effective as 2,500. Another good side effect of metformin is that most people lose a few pounds on the drug. There is a long-acting metformin on the market, but it is not quite twenty-four hours in time action. One good thing about the long-acting is that it coats the molecules of the medication to absorb more slowly, and that makes it gentler on the tummy. Some people who start metformin will have GI disturbance such as gas, diarrhea, and stomach upset. Taking it with food helps, but for most people, the problems will go away in two to three weeks. These medications are available in generic form, which makes them affordable.

If you are on the maximum dose of sulfonylurea plus metformin, what do you do if your blood glucose levels are still elevated?

PRECOSE (ACARBOSE): In 1996, a group of drugs called starch blockers came on the market. They block the effect of the enzyme that breaks down starch into glucose, so the starches are not absorbed at first. You know, eat a brownie . . . it goes away! Unfortunately, that is only part of the story. When you eat a brownie and have used one of these drugs with the first bite, it does not absorb in the first part of the small intestine. So imagine what starches do if they are not absorbed . . . they ferment. Then when they move farther down the intestine, they are absorbed. So you get all the calories plus gas.

The positive effect is that the postprandial (after-meal) blood glucose is blunted. For a high-carbohydrate meal, you don't get such a high glucose immediately after eating, and for some people, this improvement results in better blood glucose levels all around. In studies, the starch blockers resulted in about a 30 mg/dl reduction in fasting levels. The trade name of the blockers is Precose in the United States; other versions available in the United States include Migilitol (Glyset). One of the positive things about Precose is that it is not absorbed systemically, so it can be good for people who don't want to add another drug if they are already on a lot of different drugs. The downside is that they have a very modest glucose effect with lots of side effects for a high cost. This is why I rarely see a patient on one of these and I never prescribe these for my patients.

TZDS (THIAZOLIDINEDIONES): In 1997, Rezulin (troglitazone) was introduced as the first of a new class of drugs called insulin sensitizers. One of the interesting things about this drug is that the United States was the first to get it instead of the last, even though it came from Japan. As it turned out, it wasn't all that big a favor because the drug has now been linked to eighty-nine confirmed reports of liver failure, including sixty-one deaths. Consequently, on March 21, 2000, the Food and Drug Administration asked Parke-Davis, the manufacturer of Rezulin, to take it off the market. The other drugs in this class that are still available are Avandia (rosiglitazone) and Actos (pioglitazone). The group name is thiazolidinediones, or TZDs. The first group of medications that actually work at the cell-receptor level, they stimulate muscle cells to make more of the transporter substance go to the cell wall and bring the glucose into the cell. You may be asking, if these drugs work on the primary defect of type 2 diabetes, why aren't they used as first-line therapy? Studies show that Actos as monotherapy on a newly diagnosed patient can lower the HbA1C more than 2.5 points, but may cost as much as $150 a month. Currently, it is most often used as an add-on after the sulfonylurea/metformin combination has petered out. A patient can be taking as many as four medications plus insulin, so this is probably not the best way to manage diabetes and is certainly very expensive. Actos and Avandia are thought to be less likely to cause liver damage than Rezulin. But this year they made it into the spotlight when a "meta-analysis" study was done on multiple research trials using Avandia, and the author found an increase in heart disease deaths. As you can imagine, this has caused a big uproar. The FDA at this point has put in a "black box warning" in their label and is still evaluating the data from many different studies. What is a black boxed warning? It is a warning to prescribers about a particular situation with a drug that the FDA wants the reader to pay particular attention and knows that if they don't put a black box around it we could miss it in the pages and pages of stuff in the product insert. Right now, both Avandia and Actos have the same warning about congestive heart failure, but ischemic heart disease is another matter. Ischemic heart disease means you have had a clot that causes loss of blood flow to a portion of heart muscle causing it to die, also called myocardial infarction, or heart attack. That is the condition that *The New England Journal of Medicine* article accused Avandia of causing. Actos had done a large multicenter trial looking at whether Actos would improve cardiovascular risk factors and in fact they were able to show a small improvement in heart disease. The FDA will continue to evaluate all the data to explore where further warnings need to be added. There are two other cautions that should be noted for both of these drugs: (1) They both cause weight gain and fluid retention. Some people gain as much as fifty pounds. When I started Rezulin I gained twenty pounds in about six weeks. Some of it was fluid, but about fifteen pounds stayed after I stopped the drug, and it took me years to get it off; (2) Bone fractures of the arm, leg, and feet are a risk for women especially. This is different from the usual postmenopausal fractures of hip and spine. So what to do? These medications both improve blood glucose very well, but I think a person must start the protocol enlightened about potential side effects.

June and Barbara: We used to think, the more pills the merrier, but you've shined a light on the situation that shows how complicated and even confusing the choices can be and how there's an unsettling period of experimentation involved for many people. We remember our former publisher, who has type 2, was happy on metformin but tried Rezulin when it first came out. He found his blood sugars were much better on metformin, so he switched back—and incidentally saved himself a lot of money. What has been your personal experience with all the new drugs, and what combination have you settled on now?

Virginia: Right now I'm on 5 mg glipizide at bedtime and 10 mcg Byetta at meals. In the few years prior to January 2003 (see Dallas–Fort Worth epiphany, page 139) I was taking about 160 units of insulin each day to keep my A1C under 6 percent. Going on an insulin pump reduced my insulin requirement to 140 units each day, and the weight loss and Byetta has reduced my insulin to zero.

I've tried everything, including metformin before it was on the market (I got it in Germany) and I couldn't tolerate it. It did help my blood sugars, but I couldn't stay awake and I really felt bad. I tried Rezulin when it came on the market and it cut my insulin requirement in half and improved my after-meal glucose, but,

Table 2.1 • Oral Diabetes Medicines

Drug groups	Secretagogues	Biguanides	Thiazolidinediones "TZDs"	DPPIV inhibitors
Brand names (generic name) *available as generic	Diabinese (chlorpropramide*) Diabeta (glyburide*) Glucotrol or Glucotrol XL (Glipizide* or GlipizideER*)	Glucophage (Metformin*) Glucophage ER (Metformin ER*) Glucovanc—a combination of metformin and glyburide Metformin is available in combination with most other oral agents	Avandia (rosiglitazone) Actos (pioglitazone)	Januvia (sitagliptin)
Action	Increases insulin being secreted from pancreas	Decreases excess glucose from liver	Improves action of insulin on muscles making you more "sensitive" to your own insulin	Stops DPPIV from blocking effect of helper hormone—see Byetta
Caution	May cause hypoglycemia if meal is missed or exercise excessive	Side effects: 40% will have stomach upset or diarrhea, but wanes over first month. Not given to people with kidney disease, congestive heart failure, emphysema, or to binge drinkers. Watch out for lactic acidosis (flu-like symptoms)	Not given in combination with insulin. May cause weight gain, congestive heart failure	Weight neutral, no hypoglycemia unless in combo with secretagogue

Add to oral agents: Byetta: Injectable hormone (helper hormone) called an incretin mimetic—in other words, mimics a natural hormone made in the intestines. Lowers blood glucose after meals by increasing insulin production, decreases excess liver glucose, slows stomach emptying to normal, and makes you feel full sooner. Can be used in combination with sulfonylureas, metformin, or TZDs. Side effects: nausea in about 40% of people when first starting, but decreases over time. Also, most people lose weight.

alas, I fell into the small percentage of people who are allergic. For me, it caused significant swelling (my ankles looked like knees), which occurs in less than 5 percent of people. I haven't tried the new TZDs because they act the same as Rezulin and I don't want the weight gain.

June and Barbara: Should everyone who's having above-normal blood sugars try the pills?

Virginia: I know from my work with patients that there is no escaping the need for exercise and diet along with the pills or insulin or both. Insulin and pills are not a replacement for diet and exercise, they're just part of the armamentarium. Diet and exercise are still the key factors in managing type 2 diabetes.

June and Barbara: You mentioned that you took insulin in combination with pills at one time. Why is this done?

Virginia: If you're on the maximum oral agent dose and your fasting blood sugar is still too high—and therefore your blood sugar will be too high for the rest of the day (as the fasting goes, so goes the rest of the day)—some physicians will add a long-acting insulin at bedtime. By adding this dose of insulin, you can often normalize the fasting blood sugar. The pills will then work fine for the rest of the day. We call this BIDS: bedtime insulin, daytime sulfonylureas (or other oral agents). It provides a nice alternative to having to go totally onto insulin. Also in selected individuals, we use the pills and insulin in combination to avoid going to much higher doses of insulin, which could predispose the person to weight gain. In selecting a long-acting insulin, you have several choices:

NEUTRAL PROTAMINE HAGEDORN (NPH). A human insulin, both Eli Lilly and Novo Nordisk make one of these. It starts working in one to two hours, lasts eight to ten hours, and peaks in about six hours. The downside? It can cause hypoglycemia in the night when it peaks. The upside: it is cheap. The human insulins cost between $20 and $30 per vial, as opposed to about $70 per vial for analogs. Analog means they make a copy of the human insulin molecule and then move or add amino acids in different positions to change the time action of the insulin, making it either shorter-acting (Humalog, Novolog, or Apidra) or longer-acting (see below).

LANTUS (INSULIN GLARGINE). Made by Sanofi-Aventis, this is a basal insulin, which means it works to cover the baseline insulin requirement for about twenty-four hours (about 50 percent of total daily dose). It causes fewer lows than NPH.

LEVEMIR (INSULIN DETEMIR). Made by Novo Nordisk, this is a basal insulin that works for a little less than twenty-four hours but has the advantage of causing the least amount of hypoglycemia overnight and, interestingly enough, causes less weight gain than the other insulins.

June and Barbara: When is it determined that a type 2 person should go totally on insulin?

Virginia: Even though type 2 diabetes was previously called non-insulin-dependent diabetes, it's very common for type 2s to go on insulin. This makes for a lot of confusion, because as many as 25 percent to 50 percent of type 2s will eventually be using insulin to manage their diabetes. This is not something to fear. Insulin is "pure and natural" and is truly a lifesaving drug. How is this determined? Typically, people with type 2 diabetes, when diagnosed, can get along with diet and exercise. Then when their insulin production deficit becomes so large that they cannot overcome their resistance, they're given the oral agents. That works for a while. The average time that oral agents work is between five and seven years, although it can be much less time or even longer. I have a patient who has been on pills for twenty-five years. Granted, he's the only one I've seen who has made use of them that long. It's unusual, but possible.

Now let's say that you've exhausted all efforts with diet and exercise and the oral agents are no longer controlling your blood sugar in the range that you and your physician have determined to be appropriate. Probably, your fasting blood sugars are significantly over 150 and after-meal blood sugars are significantly over 200. So you are told that you should go on insulin.

June and Barbara: What happens next? How do you "go on insulin"? What kind of insulin and how much?

Virginia: There are several different ways. Some physicians will simply take you off all oral agents and start you on an insulin regimen. Others in recent years have found that if they can just get the fasting blood sugar normal, then the rest of the day will be controlled just fine with pills. They may start you on the one injection of a long-acting insulin at bedtime. The idea is that it will lower your blood sugar in the early morning hours when it ordinarily goes up because of excessive liver glucose production. This might work for a year or two before you need to add insulin coverage for meals.

If you fail on the pills, your physician may decide not to use pills at all anymore, but to go exclusively to insulin. Unit for unit, insulin may be cheaper than pills. If you're going to have to go on insulin anyway, some doctors reason, why not go straight to insulin to begin with and use insulin only? In that case, a premixed insulin may work for some people with type 2 diabetes. This means that in any dose that you draw up, 70 percent to 75 percent of the units will be NPH-type insulin (slow-acting) and 25 percent to 30 percent will be rapid-acting analog insulin or an older regular insulin. Many patients like this system because they only take two injections a day, but it does not give the patient flexibility in meal times and amount of food. If we use a premix insulin, we prefer to use one with a rapid analog instead of regular. Regular insulin takes thirty to sixty minutes to start working and lasts four to six hours, so it tends to cause more highs right after the meal and more lows four hours later. With the premix, the rapid-acting portion works for breakfast and the NPH in the middle of the day covers lunch if you don't eat too much then, but you have to eat something. That's what I meant by not a lot of flexibility. If you are the type who eats three meals a day every day at the same times, this

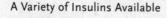

A Variety of Insulins Available

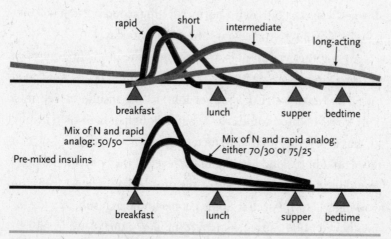

Figure 2.2 • Timing of insulin action

might be the type of regimen for you. But if you want the flexibility to eat different amounts of food at different times, you will want a basal-bolus regimen. We refer to this type of regimen as being "physiologic"; in other words, it works like your body would work if it could. So, the positive side of this type program is that it allows you to eat different amounts at different times and have flexibility in your schedule, but the downside is that it requires four to five injections a day and multiple glucose checks. Why would someone do this? Because by controlling their blood glucose better, they are less likely to have unexpected highs and lows and most of us report we feel much better. I have been accused of being "obsessive-compulsive" about managing my diabetes but I prefer to think of myself as "therapeutically self-absorbed."

On the premixed, twice-a-day regimen, many folks with type 2 diabetes will need more insulin in the evening than in the morning. This is because your insulin resistance and lack of sufficient insulin causes excessive liver glucose during the night. I tell my patients that we can't be shy about using as much insulin as it takes. The most important key for control in the type 2 on insulin is to use as much insulin as it takes to get those blood sugars down. If you start out with a normal-fasting blood sugar, it will take a lot less insulin to manage it throughout the day.

Yet another variation is to "treat only the problem" approach by using a rapid-acting insulin (Humalog, NovoLog, or Apidra) at meals and take NPH or another long-acting insulin at bedtime. This works because some type 2s have enough of their own insulin for basal coverage (baseline metabolism when not eating so that they could have good blood glucose levels if they never ate—not a good long-term solution). Now, the upside: you only have insulin working when you need it. Some people find that insulin during the day such as NPH causes them to feel hungry and they end up eating to keep up with their insulin. Oh, and it is cheap, $20 to $30 a vial. Now the downside: NPH in the evening can cause hypo-glycemia during the night. In a recent study, it was found that comparing NPH, Lantus, and Levemir, they all gave the same fasting blood glucose, but NPH causes the most hypoglycemia, and Levemir the least hypoglycemia and also the least weight gain.

June and Barbara: We notice that you've abandoned the old system of putting all type 2s on just one shot of NPH every morning. That was certainly an easy way to go, and it was June's regimen for years until she wised up and suggested to her doctor that she would like to use regular before each meal. Is the one-shot-a-day system ever used today?

Virginia: Yes, all too often type 2s are put on only one shot a day. But now, the one shot is usually Lantus at bedtime. Many physicians start people on 10 units at bed and then leave them there for months and months. We will use either Lantus or Levemir and prefer to use a formula that individualizes the dose to each person. Take your weight in pounds and divide it by 10. This will give you a dose closer to what you actually need. Then adjust the dose up or down by two to five units each week until your fasting glucose is in your target range. Unfortunately, in the United States, this has become the most common regimen and it is not getting people into good enough control. The important thing to understand if you are started on one injection a day is to test after meals as well as fasting in the morning. We have folks test after a different meal each day so that they get a full picture of how their food is affecting their glucose levels. It is important to remember that when your A1C is below 7.3, 70 percent of the contributing glucose to that A1C comes from after-meal elevations. That is why it is critical that we not only control fasting glucose, but also keep after-meal glucoses in target range as well. It is important to keep both glucose levels in the near-normal range because it just doesn't feel good for our blood glucose to swing a hundred points. Mother Nature did not design us that way. We were designed to have a blood sugar fluctuation of no more than 30 to 40 points throughout the day. If we can mimic that for people with diabetes, they feel better.

June and Barbara: There are so many kinds of insulin on the market now that a beginner might be confused when trying to buy the particular one his or her doctor has prescribed. When June started using insulin twenty-five years ago, there were few choices, because we had only animal insulins (made from the pancreases of pigs or cattle). Now, of course, the animal insulins are off the market but we have the so-called human insulins, which are exactly like the insulin the body makes. (Manufactured human insulin is made with recombinant DNA genetic engineering techniques.) Isn't it hard to explain all this to new insulin takers?

Virginia: It's not really as complicated as it sounds at first. Let's summarize. There are only five major types with different speeds of action.

1. Rapid-acting insulin, which is one of the great new inventions of diabetes care, works like we always wished regular (see number 2) would work. It actually covers the meal. You can take it right before you eat and it acts within fifteen minutes. It peaks (has its strongest effect) in sixty to ninety minutes and then goes away after about three to four hours. It has been shown to be quite effective for type 2s who lack the first-phase insulin production to cover a meal, even though they still make insulin. It is the first insulin "analog." In other words, it is made by changing the structure of the molecule to change its action instead of by adding other substances.

2. Regular is the short-acting kind that starts working in about forty-five minutes, peaks in about three hours, and is gone in five or six hours.

3. The intermediate-acting insulins are NPH, by far the most commonly used, and Lente. Lente is now off the market. NPH starts to work in thirty to ninety minutes, peaks between six and eight hours, and lasts about twelve hours.

4. The long-acting insulins are Lantus and Levemir (Ultralente is off the market). These insulins start to work in about two hours and have very little peak, more like a "swell" at ten to twelve hours, and last up to twenty-four hours. These cover basal insulin requirements, the little amount of insulin your body makes all the time, about 50 percent of your total daily insulin requirement.

5. There are several premixed combinations of NPH and regular and NPH and rapid insulin. There is the combination of 70 percent NPH and 30 percent regular insulin made by both Eli Lilly (Humulin 70/30) and Novo (Novolin 70/30). Then with the advent of the rapid-acting analogs, we have those in mixture as well. You can imagine that with my preference for rapid analogs over regular, I prefer these in the premix insulins, too. Eli Lilly came out with its premix first; to avoid any confusion with Humulin 70/30, they made the analog premix Humalog Mix 75/25. The slightly different formulation does not have any clinical significance but assures patients don't get the wrong insulin. We also have a premix Humalog Mix 50/50 which, as it implies, gives you 50 percent Humalog and 50 percent NPH. This is for patients who need a larger amount of Humalog for a larger or high-carbohydrate meal. On the other hand, when Novo came out with its analog premix they named it NovoLog Mix 70/30. As you can imagine, many mistakes are made by patients and pharmacists. I blame the FDA

for not insisting that the names be significantly different for safety. I don't feel that they have been proactive on labeling and safety issues when it comes to packaging.

Some people are still grieving the loss of animal insulins saying they can tell the difference, but in large clinical trials when the different groups don't know which insulin they are getting, there is no difference. Incidentally, there used to be another long-lasting insulin like Ultralente called PZI (protamine zinc insulin). And like Ultralente, it went off the market several years ago, but this didn't make the front pages of newspapers, because the only ones who missed it were cats with diabetes. It seems that veterinarians had found it to be the preferred insulin for cats. For several years, the poor cats were given Lantus and other long-acting insulins which didn't work as well. Recently, one of my patients told me that she has a cat with diabetes and he gets PZI U-40 (40 units per ml instead of U-100). This insulin is only available from veterinarians for cats. By the way, the cat is a really good little diabetic; if Becky has not remembered to give him the evening dose of insulin, the cat comes up to her and bumps his head against her leg to remind her to give him the insulin.

June and Barbara: Doesn't taking insulin cause people with diabetes to gain weight? You've told us that it's a powerful fat-generating hormone.

Virginia: Yes, it very well could. The person with type 2 diabetes probably has enough insulin on board but is very resistant to it. Now we add more with injections. If you think about it, if your blood sugar has been running 250 and your weight has been staying stable, it figures that a fair amount of your calories have been going out in the toilet, because the extra sugar in the bloodstream is being spilled into the urine. If we give you enough insulin to get your blood sugar down to normal, those calories that were putting sugar into your urine have to go somewhere else, right? Probably right to your thighs.

That's what I like about rapid-acting insulin at meals. Since we don't have a first-phase insulin production to cover a meal, our blood glucose gets too high immediately after eating, which stimulates a really big load of insulin later . . . much later. All this extra insulin coming in several hours after eating only makes us hungrier and makes us gain weight. Using a rapid-acting insulin in the fifteen minutes before meals replaces our first-phase insulin response so that we don't have so much second-phase insulin and, therefore, have better blood glucose levels without so much hunger and weight gain. I used Humalog before meals, with a long-acting insulin at night. I think this is an ideal regimen for type 2s who want flexibility of meal type and timing. Now that I am on Byetta and have lost a significant amount of weight, I no longer require insulin.

June and Barbara: What's the best way to teach people how to inject insulin? Do you still use an orange to practice with?

Virginia: Absolutely not! What a waste of a perfectly good orange. When a patient who needs insulin comes to me to learn how to inject, I don't talk about anything else, I just get straight to the injection procedure. I have them give themselves an injection using sterile water, so they can find out that it's not a big deal. It doesn't hurt if you do it right. Besides, the insulin syringes and pen needles are so short and fine (5 mm in length, 31 g) that you really can't feel it. Once they've done their first injection, then we can talk about other things such as managing their blood sugars.

So many people have an exaggerated fear of shots and needles that we've had to come up with innovative ways to get them over that barrier. One thing I've discovered for people with severe needle phobia is never to use an alcohol swab to prepare for the injection. The smell of alcohol sends them back to being five years old and being chased around the doctor's office by a nurse who had to hold them down to give them a shot. So no alcohol swab. Just draw up the sterile water and inject immediately. Then they can relax because they know it's nothing. They've been worried so long, now at last they're relieved.

Using alcohol on your skin is really an unnecessary waste of money, as well as cotton and alcohol. We tell people that the little germs on your skin have been buddies with your body for years, and nobody ever gets an infection from themselves. Lots of studies have been done on this. A study was even done of campers with diabetes. Can you imagine how dirty kids get? And none of them ever got an infection from their insulin shots. **Tip:** You can reuse your insulin syringes. The label on a syringe says that you should use it once and then destroy it, but that's for hospitals, since needles are never shared between patients. When I recommend to patients that they reuse their syringes, they'll ask, "How many times?" My answer is that you'll know. When it bounces off your tummy, it's time to quit using that one. Most people find that after four or five times they should switch to a new syringe.

Buying Supplies

June and Barbara: We knew one man who always used his syringes around twenty-four times. He said he actually liked them better when they got dull. We also knew an environmentally concerned woman who searched in vain everywhere for one of those old glass syringes with detachable needles. She didn't want to load the landfill with disposable syringes. She finally had to compromise by using her syringes over and over again.

We consider disposable syringes to be one of the greatest improvements in diabetes injection ease. Are there newer ways to make insulin injecting, if not pleasant, at least more convenient?

Virginia: Yes, there are many new ways to make your life much easier as far as insulin injections are concerned. A device called the insulin pen holds the insulin while you dial the dose. These pen devices are available in reusable models, which you load with a cartridge of insulin, or disposable models, which come preloaded and are disposed of when empty. Personally, I don't understand why everyone doesn't use a pen. Amazingly enough, in Europe about 95 percent of injections are given with a pen device, but in the United States it is somewhere around 25 percent. You would think that Americans would really want the high-tech solution. I think the reason is twofold. One, 80 percent of patients with diabetes are managed by primary-care physicians and they are not always familiar with all the latest gadgets because they have so many other things to stay up on, and two, we have a reimbursement system that charges patients extra if they want the pen. This is enough of a disincentive to keep them using syringes and vials.

June and Barbara: Some type 2s may be interested in the insulin infusion pumps that are advertised as the best way to get good control. We know a lot of people who gained total happiness using a pump. What's your opinion of the pump system?

Virginia: Pumps use what we call the basal-bolus insulin program. Basal refers to the insulin coverage needed to maintain blood glucose levels at times other than at meals. The bolus insulin (a concentrated dose) is used to cover meals. This schedule is designed to imitate the way your body handles its insulin output (a little bit all the time and more before meals). You don't have to be on a pump to use this system. You can use injections of long-acting insulin in the evening for a very nice basal effect and injections of rapid-acting insulin before each meal. This gives you a lot more flexibility in changing your schedule and in being able to eat more or less at different meals. You can also exercise without having an insulin peak sneak up on you. We've had a lot of success with this program. Some people call it "the poor man's pump," because syringes cost a lot less than pumps.

The cost of pumps is the reason everybody on insulin doesn't use them. It costs from $6,000 to $8,000 to get started on a pump. For those who are difficult to control, pumps are certainly a wonderful option, but most people who can manage their diabetes with exercise, oral agents, or injections see the pump as an unnecessary expense and more trouble to maintain than it's worth.

By way of example, I have one patient with type 2 diabetes who is on a pump. She has had tremendous problems controlling her blood sugar for many years. She can take neither NPH nor Lente insulins because of allergies. She could tolerate regular, but didn't like taking injections five or six times a day. She finally came to me and said, "I want a pump." On the pump, her control was greatly improved. She enjoyed the ability to eat less at some meals and more at others. She appreciated this new flexibility and ease of use.

She is a psychologist, easily the best one I've ever met. When she got her pump and started it up, she noticed it made a clicking sound. With every little basal dose it gave, it clicked. She asked how to turn off the clicks. I told her she couldn't because that's how she knew the pump was working. "The kids will go nuts over this," she said. "They're going to hate it and it's going to be distracting. This is going to be a big problem in my practice." She put the device inside an oven mitt and anything else she could find to muffle the sound. Then she started telling her young clients that she was a bionic woman and her body made clicks. They had no problem at all understanding that. It was only the parents who found her distracting. They were the ones glancing around the room with funny looks on their faces when they heard her click. By the way, she is now on a new pump that doesn't click, and she really loves it.

In my one rat study I wore a pump for about three years and really liked it. Pumps provide basal bolus insulin but with lots of tricks. The pump that I wore had a meter attached so I could test and then the result would immediately be transmitted into the pump. I would then tell the pump how much carb I was going to eat and it would calculate the dose. One great thing about a pump is that if you decide to exercise in the middle of the morning, you can't take back your Lantus, but you can tell the pump to decrease the basal insulin by 50 percent for a few hours so you don't get low from the exercise. Now we have pumps with implantable sensors that beam the results to the pump so you can see your blood glucose and the trend on the pump screen. It is one thing to see a reading of 100, but is it 100 on its way up or down? At this time the sensors are not accurate enough for the FDA to allow you to give insulin based on the number on the sensor, so people have to confirm the reading with a glucose check.

June and Barbara: People who saw the movie *Reversal of Fortune* know that the prosecution contended Claus von Bülow gave his wife a huge dose of insulin to kill her. She did not die but is in what appears to be an endless coma. Some moviegoers might have gotten the idea that insulin is a lethal drug or even a murder weapon. What are the real dangers, if any, of taking insulin, and how do you set people's minds at ease on this score?

Virginia: If you saw the movie, then you know what a bad idea it is to try to kill somebody with insulin. Granted, Sunny von Bülow is a vegetable today. However, with normal doses of insulin, the body has tremendous protective mechanisms to prevent problems from hypoglycemia. If your blood sugar starts getting too low, the pancreas starts increasing production of glucagon (the hormone that causes an increase in blood glucose; in other words, it has the opposite function of insulin). The glucagon tells the liver to start pouring out stored glucose. Eventually the body will even start breaking down muscle and fat to make sure there is enough fuel available.

Under ordinary circumstances, even when a person's blood sugar drops so low that they pass out, which is rare and virtually nonexistent in type 2s, the body uses counter-regulatory hormones such as epinephrine to generate enough glucose to protect the body and especially the brain. These mechanisms provide enough glucose to revive you. With the massive doses of insulin that Sunny von Bülow received, her brain was allowed to go without fuel long enough to be damaged.

Unlike in type 1 diabetes, type 2s have such a huge level of stored glucose in the liver that they rarely experience any hypoglycemia, let alone pass out from low blood sugar. It is possible, though, to experience the feelings of hypoglycemia, even at a higher than normal level of blood glucose, if the brain has become what we call "glucose intoxicated." This means that if you are used to running blood sugars of 300 or 400 points and we quickly bring your blood sugar down to 150 or less, you may experience the symptoms of true hypoglycemia—for example, feeling shaky, sweaty, irritable, and headachy. This happens even though your blood sugar is at or near a normal level.

If this happens to you, eat a small snack such as a few crackers. Then with a little rest, the feeling will go away. We want to avoid overtreating that pseudohypoglycemia, because what will happen is that you'll just get your blood sugar back up to 300 and you'll never adapt to normal blood sugars. If you're used to running high blood sugars, you will usually adapt to normal ones in a couple of weeks. Then you'll feel better in the long run.

June and Barbara: We've had many people come to us with the complaint that they suffer from hypoglycemia—the disease, not the hypoglycemic episodes that insulin-dependent people with diabetes sometimes experience. They're looking for books that might help them overcome the awful feelings of nervousness and depression that hypoglycemia causes. We don't know of any really good book for hypoglycemics, but we do warn them that we've heard this condition can be a precursor of diabetes. What we want to know is how is it possible to go from having a low blood sugar condition to the very reverse?

Virginia: To understand that, all you have to do is remember that many, many years before being diagnosed with diabetes, the person with type 2 diabetes lost the first-phase insulin response. If you don't have that first-phase insulin response, then when you eat a meal that is especially high in simple carbohydrates, you're going to get a real quick rise in blood glucose. This will stimulate an even bigger second-stage insulin response that in two to three hours will cause you to be hypoglycemic. We call this reactive hypoglycemia. This is the explanation of why many people tell you that they were "hypoglycemic" for years, and then eventually turned into people with type 2 diabetes, even though they seem like opposite conditions. Reactive hypoglycemia, in other words, can be one stage in the evolution of type 2 diabetes.

I have patients who say that every time they eat a candy bar or drink a Coke they feel sick. There is a simple solution to this problem: just don't do it! The diet for the person with reactive hypoglycemia is the same as for the person with diabetes. That is, eat foods high in fiber, low in sugar, low in fat—in other words, a good, healthy diet. And don't ever drink liquid sugar—meaning soft drinks or fruit juice.

June and Barbara: Is insulin a prescription drug in New Mexico? In California you don't need a prescription for some of them. How about other states?

Virginia: The older human insulins are available without prescription everywhere in the United States. This is so it will be available in case of an emergency need by a person with diabetes. Some states, though, regulate the purchase of syringes and require a prescription for a syringe. The newer analog insulins currently require a prescription, and I've been told that any new insulins approved by the FDA will also require a prescription. If you're going to be traveling, it's important that you carry your insulin with you and not check it with your luggage. When on the road it is important to carry a copy of your prescription or the pharmacy label. This will serve as proof for airport security that you are a person with diabetes and they will allow you to carry your diabetes supplies on the plane. I always advise people who are first starting on insulin to tear off the box top and put it in their purse or billfold. That way they will know the brand name and type of insulin in case they're ever out of their home area and have to buy it.

June and Barbara: Insulin in Europe is expensive like it is here. And since foreign brands have different manufacturers and names for the various types of insulin, you can really get yourself in a bind if you leave home without enough extra bottles to see you through any emergency.

Unexpected things happen when you're out of your routine and in far-off places. June once left her insulin on the seat of the airplane when arriving in Hawaii. Fortunately, she called the airport and they held it for her even though she was silly enough not to have her name on the case in which she was carrying it. Another time her regular insulin clouded up in France (the clouding was caused by silicon from repeated needle insertions into the bottle and was harmless, but she didn't know that). Then she had the experience of buying an insulin of a different strength (U40 instead of U100) and had to do complex calculations to get the correct dosage. Let her foolishness be a lesson to you (although all insulins are now the same strength abroad as here).

Since many diabetes supplies—insulin, pills, test strips—have expiration dates, how many weeks' or months' supply should a person buy? You don't want to run out, but you also don't want to let expensive products expire. There must be some way to be safe but not sorry when you look in your medicine chest.

Virginia: When insulin is manufactured, it will have at least a two-year expiration date marked on the bottle. So the farthest out you can get insulin is usually a two-year expiration date, but one-year expiration from the time you purchase it should be more than adequate. You probably only need to keep a month's supply. Since the insulin you purchase from the drugstore has been carefully refrigerated, you'll want to keep your spare bottles in the refrigerator, too. (The insert in the insulin package says, "Insulin should be stored in a cold place, preferably in a refrigerator.") The insulin you are currently using can be kept at room temperature, and it can be kept for a month that way. If you're one of those people who don't use up a bottle in a month, I would suggest keeping it in the fridge and taking it out about an hour before you're going to use it. If you use it up in two or three weeks, leaving it at room temperature is no problem. (By the way, the inside of your car is not considered room temperature.)

Most syringes have an expiration date, but as long as they haven't been contaminated they're probably just fine.

June and Barbara: What do you mean by contaminated? We've never heard of that.

Virginia: Let's say you found them in the garage in storage and you see that years ago they got wet and have been chewed on by mice—you'd want to dispose of those syringes. If they're still in their plastic bag or wrapper and have not had their protective covers removed and have not been through an atomic bomb attack, they should be okay.

June and Barbara: So far June's syringes have survived a number of California earthquakes. But unlike syringes, pills can get out of date, can't they?

Virginia: Yes, oral agents usually have an expiration date, but that date is usually several years out, so that's no problem. The real problem with stocking up on any medication too far ahead is that if for some reason your physician should decide that you need to change the medication regimen, you're stuck with these drugs; you can't take them back. Could you use oral agents beyond the expiration date? Probably, but the pharmacists won't tell you that it's okay. I would talk to my doctor about this.

June and Barbara: How about test strips? Sometimes people buy a lot of them at once to get a better price, and then they find them going out of date.

Virginia: Test strips are the one item to be careful with. They do go bad. I would watch the expiration date and I would not buy any strips whose date is not at least six months away. Granted, you would probably use them up before a slightly earlier expiration date, but it's best to be on the safe side. Strips are very fragile and very sensitive to moisture or excessive heat. If left in the heat or the cold, in the car, or with the lid off the bottle—especially in the damp atmosphere of a bathroom—they can be damaged. The meter companies have now come up with advanced ways to calibrate the meter so that the meter knows when the strips expire and won't let you use expired strips.

June and Barbara: *Diabetes Forecast* publishes a Buyer's Guide to Diabetes Products each year in its January issue. It's a detailed listing and description of all products of all kinds, from carrying cases to insulin pumps to medical IDs. At the end is a complete list of manufacturers and suppliers with their addresses and toll-free numbers. How helpful do you find this information, and what's the best way to use it?

Virginia: The problem with this information is that there is no evaluation of the products. They list junk meters right up there equally with the quality meters. Therefore, there is no way to compare the products. Do I find this guide helpful? Maybe a little. I already know the manufacturers' toll-free numbers, but I guess for some people this may be a place to call and ask questions. I wish *Consumer Reports* would do an article giving a qualitative analysis of the different meters. Short of waiting for that to happen, you can always ask your diabetes educator, who has probably had more experience with all these products than any other single person and can help you decide on the best product for you.

June and Barbara: Actually *Consumer Reports* finally did an evaluation of meters in the October 1996 issue. At the time, there were twenty-one different models on the market, but they tested only eight. They reported: "All meters we tested provided results that were accurate enough to be used with confidence." In their ratings, the Glucometer Elite (Bayer) and the One Touch (LifeScan) came out number one and number two. Since then, however, so many new meters and upgraded models have come onto the market that there would probably be different winners. Check with your diabetes educator for the latest meter information.

What do you think of mail-order sources for purchasing supplies and equipment? About ten different ones in different states advertise each month in the Shopper's Guide section at the back of *Diabetes Forecast*. Others send out catalogs and newsletters. Have many of your patients used these services and found them advantageous?

Virginia: Some people do like them because they don't have to drive around town to find things. Having supplies delivered right to your door saves time. But often the prices of the mail-order supplies are similar to the prices at the discount houses in your town, and buying locally saves you the cost of shipping, handling, and delivery (although if you're dealing with an out-of-state mail-order house, you can save the sales tax). I'd say it's a toss-up. Some people like mail-order sources, others don't find them to be advantageous. My biggest complaint with the mail-order places is that they often change your meter. They send you a few months' worth of your strips and then a letter saying they are sending you a new free meter, and people think this is a good deal. What it is is an inferior meter made in a foreign country and is not very accurate but more profitable for the mail-order business.

3

Exercise

Your Lifetime Savings Plan

IN HER BOOK *MAKING THE MOST OF YOUR MONEY*, PERSONAL finance expert Jane Bryant Quinn advises that for lifetime financial security you should always "pay yourself first." By this she means that out of whatever dollars you make each month you should set aside 10 percent for saving before you do anything else with your money. Our advice for exercise is the same as hers for money. Before you plan anything else in your day, set aside 10 percent of your available time for exercise—for most of us that will average out at thirty to ninety minutes. Ms. Quinn is adamant that financial investment should be regular and inviolable; you should never say, "There's something I'd rather do with my money right now. I'll skip saving this month and double the amount next month." And we're adamant that exercise should be regular and inviolable; you should never say, "There's something I'd rather do with my time today. I'll skip my exercise and do twice as much tomorrow." The reason for both rules is that the saving and the exercise have to be a routine, a habit, and if you break the routine once, it's easier to break it the next time . . . and the next . . . and the next, until you wake up one morning and find yourself in deep financial or physical trouble.

Ms. Quinn advocates different kinds of investments for different people. Some people aren't comfortable with the gyrations of the stock market and prefer mutual funds or the even more secure and stable money market accounts and T-bills. Some don't like the trouble of handling rental property, while others are willing to expend effort on property management in exchange for income and tax advantages. She even suggests a variety of investments for the same person to create a balanced savings portfolio and to avoid the risk of putting all your financial eggs in one basket.

We feel the same way about exercise. Some people like to play tennis, some enjoy square dancing, hiking, skating, walking, swimming, or skiing. Although most people don't or can't invest the time and effort it takes to run marathons, there are those who believe it's worth all the tremendous exertion in exchange for the mind and body benefits they derive from training and running in them. We also think that a balanced exercise portfolio is a good idea. Combining something that's aerobic with some strength training and possibly a competitive sport will give you activities to see you through all weather, seasonal, and personal mood fluctuations and will condition all parts of your body.

It's not easy to adhere to your savings program when you see others blowing their money on clothes or cars or vacations whenever they feel like it, with not a thought in the world for their economic futures. And it's not easy to stick to your exercise program when you're awash in a sea of workaholics who grind away fourteen hours a day and couch potatoes whose major exercise is reaching for a bowl of potato chips or punching buttons on the TV remote.

But the rewards are there for both Ms. Quinn's plan and ours. If you religiously follow her counsel, you will be able to accumulate amazing wealth in a lifetime. You will be financially comfortable and secure when others about you are desperately floating loans or filing for bankruptcy or moving in with relatives. If you religiously follow our counsel, it's amazing the health you will be able to enjoy for your lifetime. You will be youthfully vigorous and vital when your contemporaries are sluggish and bloated and old before their time. On top of that, our plan has a big dividend, one that's as good in terms of your health as winning the lottery would be in terms of your wealth: your diabetes will be in good control.

And here's the best part: both these plans—the saving and the exercise—that are so beneficial for your well-being can evolve into a joy and a pleasure if you enter into the spirit and make a challenging game of them.

We'll leave it up to Ms. Quinn and others to put you on the road to a lifetime money-saving program. We're here to put you on the road to a lifetime health-saving program and help you put your best foot forward.

—June and Barbara

Benefits of Exercise

June and Barbara: Virginia, you must be aware that both of us are exercise fanatics. We'll bet, though, that you didn't know we've written three entire books about sports—one on downhill skiing, one on cross-country skiing, and one on bicycling. And in 1977, with the help of 158 exercise enthusiasts who have diabetes, we published the first book ever to deal solely with exercise therapy for diabetes: *The Diabetic's Sports and Exercise Book: How to Play Your Way to Better Health*. Then, in 1995 we did an update of the book, changing the title to the more politically correct *The Diabetes Sports and Exercise Book*. We were happy to collaborate with Claudia Graham, who has a Ph.D. in exercise science and a master's degree in public health and is a certified diabetes educator. But her best credentials are that she has diabetes and is a near fanatic (like us!) when it comes to exercise. We learned a lot from her, much of which we'll pass on to you here.

Another thing we learned was how our exercise enthusiasts with diabetes had fared over eighteen years since the first edition of that book. Of course we couldn't track them all down. Many had moved and many of the women had changed their names. Even so, we found enough to make us more convinced than ever that sports and exercise have ongoing, health-producing benefits for people with diabetes. And it's not just physical health. From the upbeat, positive attitudes they exhibited in their responses, it was easy to see that their mental health was in as great shape as their bodies.

We still feel just as passionate about the value of exercise for people with diabetes as we did then. And more than ever, we keep preaching that others should become as fanatic about exercise as we are. Now that we've revealed our prejudice up front, we'll ask you how you rank exercise as a part of diabetes treatment.

Virginia: Probably when the whole truth is known, it will turn out that exercise is the most important component in diabetes control. Once again, I go back to the idea of living like our ancestors: being very physically active and eating a low-fat, high-fiber diet.

June and Barbara: Since this is a totally honest book, we must reveal that you didn't always believe that exercise is the most important component in keeping diabetes in control—or, rather, even though you believed it, you didn't put it into practice yourself. As one of the author Leo Buscaglia's wisest teachers said to him, "To know and not to do is not to know." So we hope you will forgive us if we take a brief trip down memory lane with some quotes from your very own pen to show what the ghost of Virginia past said about exercise:

> Frankly, exercise is the hardest thing for me to get a grip on. I know that when we find the gene for type 2 diabetes, he will be stretched out on his back with his feet up. I've not met one type 2 who loves to exercise. It's a constant battle for us to get out and hoof it down the road even though it's a vital part of keeping our diabetes in control. I constantly battle with myself to get out there and get moving. When other people talk about how good exercise feels, I wonder if there's some genetic reason that we type 2s don't get addicted to it. Is it related to the fact that we don't use glucose the same way "normal" people do?

Then in 2003 something happened to Virginia. Something momentous. Something life changing. We call it "the miracle of the Dallas/Fort Worth airport." It was there that Virginia experienced an epiphany. She was returning home from a conference and, well, we'll let her tell you how she lived it on page 138 (Transition Time).

June and Barbara: Now we want to make a little philosophical statement. We think every nurse and doctor—and every person with diabetes—should cease calling exercise a prescription, as in the question, "What is your exercise prescription?" or "This is your exercise prescription for the first month." Don't ever think of exercise as a prescription—some kind of bitter pill to swallow for your own good. Think of it as an opportunity to have fun, to go out, and play the way you did as a kid.

Now, having put you in the right frame of mind, we can show you what exercise can do for you and how to get yourself doing it.

Exercise makes everything about diabetes therapy easier. It makes it easier to:

- Control your blood sugar;
- Lose weight;
- Keep fit in the cardiovascular sense;
- Lower your blood fats;
- Increase your muscle strength and flexibility;
- Deter the "inevitable" process of aging;
- Avoid complications;
- Keep your spirits high and enhance your appearance and self-esteem.

Virginia: As a health professional, I concur with your entire list. I might add that the most important thing exercise does for overweight type 2s is to change their metabolism so that they burn more calories even if they're sitting still. The books that explain this phenomenon best are those by Covert Bailey, who first published his *Fit or Fat?* in 1977, and since then *The New Fit or Fat* as well as *The Fit or Fat Target Diet, The Fit or Fat Target Recipes,* and *The Fit or Fat Woman*. What he says, over and over again, is that "the ultimate cure for obesity is exercise."

June and Barbara: Yes, we've been preaching the Covert Bailey gospel since he came out with his first book. What people loved about his program was that initially he recommended a total of only twelve minutes of continuous aerobic exercise three times a week. That's not much time to give up for so much in return. Have you had any patients who have used the Covert Bailey program and found it helped them lose weight and significantly improve their diabetes control?

Virginia: Yes. Lois is a patient of mine who has the enviable life of spending half the year in Albuquerque and the other half on a lake in Michigan. (You get to guess which half where.) She has done an incredible job of managing her diabetes with exercise and diet. My educator partner, LaVerne, first started working with Lois while she was on insulin. With daily exercise Lois was able to lose fifty pounds and now has perfect blood sugars with no medications. She enjoys hosting in her home students who come to Michigan for music camp, including my daughter, Melanie, who says, "Lois is rad." (Lois has published two books of her wonderful recipes.)

So it's agreed, exercise makes all our diabetes goals easier to achieve, but how can you make exercise itself easier?

Setting Goals

June and Barbara: You just start exercising. To begin, take whatever baby steps you have to—even if you exercise only four or five minutes a day. Thinking about exercising is what's hard. If you start doing something—almost anything—you're on your way. You've probably heard the saying, "Appetite comes with eating." Well, motivation to exercise comes with exercising.

Of course, there are some strategies and tricks you can use to get you going and keep you at it. The first is to block out a time slot. Any time is great, though some experts especially recommend walking after meals. Back when we were working long hours in the SugarFree Center, the only way we could get in our exercise on weekdays was to do it right after breakfast. June did a half hour on a Schwinn Aerodyne (which provides both arm and leg exercise), and Barbara did thirty minutes of aerobics on a trampoline. On the weekends, we would bike or walk. Now that we work out of our home office and aren't tied down to an 8:00 a.m. to 5:00 or 6:00 p.m. schedule (we can just work all the time, weekends and holidays included), we still try to exercise first thing in the morning right after breakfast, usually around 6:00 a.m. June does stretching and at least twenty minutes on her new semirecumbent bike; it has a chairlike back so she can read or write while cycling and the time just races by. Barbara does stretching and either the Exercycle or the treadmill. We both work out with hand weights (June at five pounds and Barbara at eight) to keep the upper body strong enough for us to be able to lift our luggage into the overhead compartment in airplanes—a top priority for us. We consider ourselves lucky to have an upstairs office so we have a kind of natural StairMaster workout. Then in the late afternoon either or both of us may take a thirty- to forty-five-minute neighborhood walk.

We used to go to a gym, but as it grew increasingly crowded (they kept offering membership specials), we bailed out in favor of home workouts.

What we're trying to emphasize here is that you should work out your time schedule to fit your own life and sports activities. Everyone can do it. If you have to cut down on your time reading the newspaper or chatting on the telephone or playing bridge or watching TV, that's what you have to do.

Actually, cutting down on TV watching is one of the best

things you can do for yourself. A *New York Times* article told of a study by psychologist Robert Klesges of Memphis State University. He discovered that when children watch television, "they lapse into a deeply relaxed, almost semiconscious state . . . between resting and sleeping." This lowers their metabolic rate so that these children burn fewer calories watching TV than they would if they sat still doing nothing and almost as few as if they were sleeping. This may contribute to the increase in type 2 diabetes in children and young people.

Dr. Klesges believes that this TV-induced drop in metabolic rate could be a major contributor to the increasing evidence of obesity in this country. In other words, it's the opposite of Covert Bailey's exercise-induced revving up of the metabolism. So cut down on TV time. It will prevent softening of the body as well as softening of the brain.

But whatever other activity you have to give up, just don't chicken out with that tired old excuse, "I have no time for exercise."

Many people may be reluctant to get going with exercise because they have no specific goals. Nothing is accomplished if you don't figure out beforehand exactly what it is that you want to accomplish. So here's our pitch on goals.

Set Short-term Goals by the Week

Your goal must be specific, concrete, and realistically ambitious. (You can read about the art of setting goals in our book *Psyching Out Diabetes*, written with psychologist, Dr. Richard Rubin.) A main point to remember is that the goal must be one you really want to reach. It won't work to let your spouse or even your doctor set your goal. If you set it, you're much more likely to accomplish it. It's okay to let your friends and family know your goal, as they may be able to help you stick with it.

Don't Set Your Goals too High

This is another of the basic rules of goal setting. If you're thinking of jogging, for instance, you begin with half-mile runs, and then eventually you might want to work up to something as grandiose as five miles per week and in a few years twenty miles per week. All the new books on exercise emphasize that you should start out slow; the more out of shape you are, the slower you should start out. In fact, we've heard that to get in shape, it takes a month for every year you've been out of shape. For some of us, that adds up to quite a chunk of time.

Have a Do-It-Every-Day Goal

For people with diabetes, it is preferable to have the goal of exercising every day rather than the usual three or four times a week idea that has been so prominent in health advice. This is because it's easier to balance your medication and adjust your diet with daily activity. (There are exceptions, which we will explain.) One excellent walking program, *Walking Off Weight*, by Robert Sweetgall, Roba Whiteley, and Robert Neeves, advocates an eight-days-a-week goal, and that means walking not only every day but also sometimes twice in one day so that if you miss a day occasionally, you'll still have done seven workouts a week.

Covert Bailey, who several years ago was preaching his twelve minutes of aerobic exercise three times a week as a total program, has switched to new advice: "Exercise longer, not harder." He has learned that his original method of having people use the formula 220 minus their age to get their maximum heart rate to set their exercise target zone is not effective for about 30 percent of the population and was causing a lot of people to overdo or underdo. (Approximately 15 percent of people have a slower heartbeat than

the average, and 15 percent have a faster heartbeat.) Now he emphasizes that "exercising at low levels is far, far more beneficial than we
originally thought." One of his new rules is to "exercise as much as
possible." And he's recommending that even beginners exercise six
times a week for twelve minutes.

We might sum up by saying that your goal should be to try to
get some exercise every day, even if it's only a few minutes and
done in more than one short session. (See how reasonable we are?)
Cardiologist James Rippe, director of the University of Massachu-
setts Medical School Exercise Physiology Lab, says: "You don't
have to turn your life upside down to do things that have a profound impact on how happy, productive, and healthy you are." He
recommends a simple two-step plan to feel better and reduce risk
of heart disease: (1) Eat cereal with skim milk for breakfast, then (2)
go out for a fifteen-minute walk. This simple plan works just as well
for people with diabetes.

Virginia: It will be a relief for many people to know they don't
have to aim for exercises that leave them sweating and panting
and exhausted. Do you have any more such motivators in your
gym bag?

June and Barbara: We always have more. To impress yourself with
your spectacular progress in fulfilling your goals, keep records, or as
the sports people call it, a logbook. These records can be as simple
as jotting down the day of the week, the time of day, the kind of exercise, and the length of time you exercised. You can use an ordinary
monthly calendar with large squares for each day. Or, if you keep
blood sugar and medication records, in one of the logbooks provided by meter companies, add your exercise record to this.

At the end of each week, total your time and see if you achieved your goal or how close you came to it. Maybe you even surpassed your goal and you can crow about it.

Virginia: That's easy enough. When do you get to the hard part?

June and Barbara: There really isn't any hard part—except in certain people's minds. What we're coming to now is the easiest part—the reward or celebration for achieving your goal. We have a friend who has this down to a science. She has a reward not every week, month, or year, but every day. This is the way it works: it's two miles from her house to a neighborhood coffeehouse, a vendor of freshly roasted choice gourmet coffee beans that features outstanding cups of coffee, cappuccinos, and espressos and the owner's own fresh, home-baked fruit muffins (low in sugar and moderate in size). She takes her blood sugar—it's usually low after the two-mile walk—and then she's eligible for the reward: coffee and a blueberry, cherry walnut, or peach muffin, or whatever is in season. The muffin—or sometimes half of one—is just enough fuel to sustain her for the return trip.

So all you do is find a spot that's far enough away, a spot with something good to drink and/or eat, and take off. If you don't live in a coffeehouse-filled area as our friend's or don't like coffee or tea, you can carry your reward in your backpack and sit and enjoy it at the midpoint of your walk. This is just one idea. There are many nonfood rewards—even such schemes as putting 10 cents in a piggy bank for every mile or minute you walk. This is also a good way of keeping track of how long you exercise each day. The money saved this way is, of course, a discretionary fund to spend in any wild and crazy and impractical way you choose.

There are probably some saintly people out there who don't even crave such material rewards. Their reward is the inner satisfaction of achieving their goal and feeling healthier and more energetic, looking better, and enjoying life more.

Stretching

Virginia: You're right about the importance of goals. Almost all successful people work with goals and rewards. Now the next question that comes to mind is, what kinds of exercise do you consider best for type 2s?

June and Barbara: No matter when, where, or what kind of exercise you're doing, you should always begin with stretching. This increases flexibility and helps prevent injuries in whatever activity you follow it up with. Barbara even found stretching had curative powers. To "celebrate" June's twenty-fifth diabetes anniversary, we did what is known as *wanderjahr*. When German students finish college they often take a year off for travel. We didn't take a year off, but we traveled a lot: Hong Kong, Bali, Wyoming, Paris, Florence, Switzerland, plus a number of local trips. Wherever we went, Barbara carried a heavy bag full of cosmetics and diabetes supplies, including food for emergency situations, on her shoulders. When the year was over, Barbara's back was so stiff and painful from being thrown out of alignment by that bag she could hardly swing her legs out of bed in the morning. On her orthopedist's advice she started a program of stretching exercises. She also put a bowl of rice and chalk under her bed beneath the area where the pain was greatest. This was something she'd read in a book about Chinese medicine. In a few months the pain went away, never to return again. (She still stretches every morning and the chalk and rice remain under her bed just in case that had something to do with the cure.)

Claudia Graham provides some good stretching tips in *The Diabetes Sports and Exercise Book*. For almost all stretches it's best to stretch slowly to the limit of regular joint motion. Stop when you feel resistance, before you feel any pain. Hold the stretch for about twenty seconds, because when the muscle is first stretched, the nerve impulses signal the muscle to contract (it thinks it's being overstretched). When you hold for twenty seconds, those nerve impulses go away, the muscle relaxes, and you have a greater and less painful stretch.

People are not rubber bands. Too-aggressive stretching (rapid bouncing and twisting) can cause injury. Always perform a more progressive, nonballistic stretch. Cold muscles resist stretching, so some warm-up activity is a good idea. Always stretch before vigorous exercise, as well as afterward to prevent sore muscles. It makes a lot of sense to stretch daily and to incorporate stretches into your regular exercise program.

A few words of caution: If you're out of shape, have limited hip flexibility, or have a history of back problems, check with your doctor first. If you have proliferative retinopathy, you may need to modify some of these stretches. Once you have gotten the go-ahead from your doctor, remember these tips:

- Pay close attention to technique.
- Never bend from your waist by rounding your back.
- Bend at the hips and knees while keeping your back straight.
- Don't hold your breath while bending, because that can cause a rise in blood pressure. It's best to exhale as you stretch.
- Proceed slowly and hold for twenty to thirty seconds. If it hurts at all, let up on the stretch.
- Do a warm-up activity before stretching. Even a hot shower will help.

You need to stretch different muscle groups depending upon your exercise activity. But this is only an introduction to Stretching 101, so we recommend an excellent book by Bob Anderson, titled *Stretching*, with examples for every sport.

At first, stretch four times with a rest between repetitions. Try to do each stretch at least three to four times a week. It may take you a while, but by initiating your stretches for a few seconds, eventually you'll be able to hold a stretch for twenty seconds.

Virginia: It appears that stretching exercises are themselves a mini-workout. I also like the cat's way: one nice stretch upon waking. But I do see the logic of Claudia's stretching exercises, and warmed-up muscles are necessary for launching into the more strenuous activity that we always recommend at the Diabetes Network—aerobic exercise that benefits people with diabetes in particular. By aerobic, I mean an activity that is continuous and rhythmic and done at a level that feels somewhat difficult. This means walking, jogging, running, bicycling, rowing, swimming, jumping rope, aerobic dancing, roller-skating, and treadmill-walking.

June and Barbara: Aerobic is the word, all right. And you've given us the main choices, except maybe cross-country skiing, which is the most intensive workout of all. Your selection of sport is controlled to some extent by where you're going to be exercising: at home, in your neighborhood, or in a fitness center or gym. The aerobic possibilities in each of these locations differ.

In Your Home

If you can't leave the house because of weather, small children, hazardous neighborhood, or physical problems, then your exercise will depend largely on in-house equipment. You buy what you like and what you can afford. We've mentioned trampolines and jumping ropes, both inexpensive but quite intensive. More pricey (in order of least expensive to most expensive) are rowing machines, cross-country skiing machines, Exercycles, treadmills, and stair-climbing machines. A good treadmill can set you back a pretty penny, say, $1,200 to $3,000. The popular stair-climbers or step machines cost up to $5,000. (June's orthopedist warns against the stair-climbers because they're too hard on the knees.) **Thrift tip:** Sad to say, many people in the first throes of exercise enthusiasm rush out and buy expensive equipment. Then when the thrill is gone and the equipment is gathering dust or becomes a place to hang clothes, they sell everything at a drastically reduced price. Look for ads in your local newspaper. You can find terrific bargains there. And however you get your equipment, you won't let your exercise enthusiasm wane and allow the equipment to gather dust or become a clothes rack, will you? No, of course not!

In judging equipment, you have to be certain that you aren't going for something that will stress your back or your bad elbow or whatever other physical injuries or debilities you may have. There's a lot to think about, so be wary of fast-talking salespeople who are themselves athletic types and don't understand that all of us are not as young and/or in as prime physical condition as they are.

Last there is the gentlest, least-damaging exercise of them all, swimming. If your house already has a pool, fine. If not, prepare for an investment of something like the equivalent of a first-class trip around the world or the purchase of a new Mercedes.

If you do have access to a pool, there's a new swimming pool exercise we recently heard about: water walking, which means walking in the pool. The resistance of the water multiplies the effectiveness of your exercise. June did a lot of this when she went to a rehab center for her shattered tibial plateau (caused by slipping on a pool of butter while making an omelet). It was very instrumental in her recovery.

In Your Neighborhood

Neighborhood exercise choices include walking on sidewalks and in malls, jogging, biking, and, for those who live in snowy country, cross-country skiing in winter. You can also look for a public swimming pool in your neighborhood. Some condo complexes allow nonresidents to use their pools for a membership fee.

Virginia: Or you could build a house with an indoor pool and a treadmill in the water . . . can you believe it? I have a friend here in Albuquerque who is building such a house, in which you will be able to look at the mountains while walking on the treadmill in the water. Okay, most of us will never be able to afford it.

In a Fitness Center or Gym

June and Barbara: Almost all modern fitness centers have aerobic exercise available as well as weights and Nautilus-style machines for muscle-strengthening exercises. At the LA Fitness gym, where we used to go, the trainers want you to warm up for at least twenty minutes on the aerobic equipment before you begin your strength-training workout. Not a bad idea, because a little of each is always better than a lot of either.

The advantage of the gym is that you can go in any weather and do a variety of exercises; the disadvantage is that at certain hours, especially early mornings and evenings, the gym is overcrowded and you have to waste time waiting to use the equipment. Ask the attendants which hours are the least busy and see if you can work your schedule around those times.

The other leading disadvantage is the cost. The initial fee can be as low as free if the company is running an advertised special or it could be up to $150. There is a monthly charge of maybe $25 to $50, depending on your neighborhood (obviously, high-rent areas will charge the most); often family members can sign on together for lower rates. Be sure to investigate the company, as lots of scammy stuff goes on with some of these chains. The gym may go out of business after you've paid a big up-front fee, or it may sell out to another organization that won't honor your initial contract.

Now comes the big decision. You've picked your main workout location, so which particular sports are you going to go for?

Here are some guidelines:

- Pick the exercises that most appeal to you.
- Choose the exercises you can do most often.
- Select more than one exercise, especially if you're older, so that you can alternate them and give different muscles time to recoup between sessions.
- Do aerobic exercise, but add some form of muscle-strengthening exercise. Sixty-five percent of the body's muscles are above the hips and most aerobic exercises do little to strengthen them.
- Choose some load-bearing exercise. For example, if swimming is your main thing, also do some activity in which you're on your feet. This is especially important for women because it helps avoid osteoporosis.

Walking: Shoes and Socks

Virginia: That sounds like an ideal plan, but you know many of us will be lucky to get into one form of exercise. And some of us type

2s need a little extra nudge to put us on the right track. Could you give us at least a hint about which exercise would be the easiest and least likely to defeat us in the beginning?

June and Barbara: That's exactly what we were hoping you would ask. The answer is clear and unequivocal: walking. To quote the (albeit somewhat prejudiced) author of a book on walking, Casey Meyers, "walking is the most injury-free, sustainable, effective, complete exercise" there is. He also claims it uses more energy and burns more calories than running. Furthermore, Meyers proves via research that humans are biomechanically engineered to be walkers, not runners. As he puts it, "if God had meant humans to run, He would have given us the locomotion system of a horse."

Walking's our all-time favorite. Though we do other sports off and on, walking is the activity we've most successfully woven into the fabric of our lives. It's a low-impact, lifetime exercise. You can do it fast (four miles an hour) or slow (two miles an hour). It's quick, convenient, and inexpensive. You can do it alone, with one other person, or in a group. Group and individual mall walking programs are now available for people of all ages in some shopping centers. In our neighborhood, there are two walking tracks in two parks, and we see people out doing their fitness walks at all hours of the day (except when it's 100 degrees outside and smoggy).

Walking is also a perfect vacation sightseeing activity. On our *wanderjahr* we spent ten days walking all over Florence and two weeks walking streets and roads and trails in the area around Montreux, Switzerland.

Walking is the least expensive exercise, especially compared to such facility-and-equipment-intensive sports such as golfing, tennis, and skiing. But there are a couple of things you do have to invest a bit of money in: shoes and socks. For a person with diabetes, choosing these isn't exactly a simple matter. We say this because of the amount of attention that must be paid to the legendary "diabetic foot." You find long lists of dos and don'ts about foot care in all diabetes manuals. We were surprised when one of our own books was indexed with a heading "diabetic foot," because no other part of the diabetic person's body was so listed. There was no entry for the diabetic thumb or ear. It's as if when you have diabetes, your Achilles' heel is a whole Achilles' foot. Can you explain why diabetic feet are different from ordinary feet?

Diabetic Feet

Virginia: Actually, diabetic feet start out like normal feet but suffer the effects of the disease as time goes by. When glucose levels stay above normal—over 180 to 200—year after year, two different problems add up to serious changes in the feet.

The first problem is the decrease in circulation that can occur because of diabetes. Excess glucose works to plug up your blood vessels. Poor circulation in your feet and legs means that they can't respond to the stress of a little sore by combating germs and infections. Your feet cannot heal the way normal feet do.

The second problem is the damage to nerves that high blood sugar can cause. When the nerves serving your feet and legs are damaged, they act like a faulty electrical circuit. First, you get static—tingling, strange shooting pains—and eventually numbness. This may seem like a relief after the tingling and pain, but it's very dangerous because you don't know when you're getting the kind of excessive pressure that causes blisters, or you may be unaware that you've stepped on a tack. Eventually you could end up with structural deformities of the foot, because it is the nerves that keep the muscles stimulated to hold your feet in shape.

THE FRENCH CONNECTION

On the subject of nerve damage we have a tale to tell. We call it "the French Connection." Fortunately, it has a happy ending.

There's a little restaurant in our neck of the Los Angeles woods named Le Petit Jacques. It's named after the owner, a Napoleon-size Frenchman. We often go there with friends. His charming wife works there off and on. One night when we saw her, she looked very bad. Barbara asked her what was the matter, and she said she just found out she has diabetes. She discovered this when she went to the doctor because she was having such pain in her feet. At any rate, she didn't know that we had anything to do with diabetes, but a friend—a nurse—who was dining with us told her we had written several books on the subject. We offered to bring her a book that might help her. I guess we all know which book *that* would be—the earlier edition of the book you're now reading. We delivered it the following day.

Every time we went there we always looked for her, but she was nowhere to be seen. When we asked Petit Jacques how she was getting along, his response was a Gallic shrug. Not a good sign.

But a couple of months later, when for another visit to the restaurant, lo, Mme Petit Jacques was on the scene. And this time she was radiant! We told her how wonderful she looked and she allowed as how she *felt* wonderful. When we asked her how her feet were, she smiled and said, "They're fine now. The doctor gave me something and it really worked."

"What did he give you?" She said something that we couldn't quite understand (a petit accent problem) but it was something that sounded like Levenet (?!). Mme Petit Jacques said she was supposed to take it three times a day, but since it made her too dopey to work she took it upon herself (as patients are wont to do) to reduce the dosage to once a day, and it still seemed to do the job. When June asked her how her blood sugars were, she very professionally rattled them off. They were all right on the money.

She was so happy that she gave us each a complimentary dessert, which was outstanding—and not too sweet.

And so, Virginia, oracle of diabetes medications, what might that magic potion that drove away her pain be? We don't think it was one of the capsaicin persuasion since we're familiar with those.

Virginia: What a sad story at Le Petit Jacques. I'm happy it turned out all right. The sad part is that about 14 percent of people already have neuropathy at the time of their diagnosis. In fact that's often what initially drives them to the doctor.

As for the "magic potion," it sounds as if she's taking Lyrica. Here is the rundown on that as well as other neuropathy drugs.

The old-time drug that is our standby (meaning inexpensive) is amitriptyline. It's an antidepressant that actually helps some, but its side effects are bothersome—dry mouth, some weight gain. (Just what we don't need!) We have patients take it at night because of its sleep effect.

Then the next step is to use gabapentin (Neurontin), which is an antiseizure drug but helps with nerve pain. In studies, it has the same effectiveness as amitriptyline but has fewer side effects.

Next up the line is Lyrica. It's in the same general class as Neurontin, but seems to work better, has fewer side effects, and is not as tricky to adjust the dose.

We are also using Cymbalta for neuropathic pain. It is an antidepressant and sort of related to Prozac, but is a serotonin and norepinephrine reuptake inhibitor. The norepinephrine part is what makes it both an effective depression drug and a help with nerve pain. My experience with Cymbalta is that for severe pain it may be the best *if* it works. About half of those who try it love it, others don't find it helpful.

Interestingly, none of these drugs treat the underlying damage, they only deal with pain. Two classes of drugs may actually deal with the pathology, but neither has been approved by the FDA. This is an extremely difficult issue to prove in clinical trials. There is no objective measure of improvement (the patient having less pain does not move the FDA). One is the aldose reductase inhibitor group. Scientists have been studying them for years and many of the drugs have gone up in flames due to side effects before they made it to market. There are several still in the pipeline. We will have to wait to see if they make it.

June and Barbara: Obviously this is why diabetic feet need special loving care. And that's the reason we're going to go into detail about purchasing shoes and socks. Not that everyone—with diabetes or not—who is an avid walker or jogger shouldn't be concerned about choosing the right foot attire. You can't enjoy walking unless your feet feel good both during and after. And it's not easy to make your selection these days, since there is a proliferation of walking and running shoes and all the major brands have some new technology to hype. Something new comes along every day, and the buyer has to be wary.

Not only is there controversy about all this fancy technology, but there is also little agreement about whether you should buy shoes designed specifically for walking or shoes specifically designed for running. We personally go for running shoes, since the tread is usually more pronounced and therefore cushions and grips better. Robert Sweetgall says you should make sure that the shoes do not have flat bottoms. They should have a rocker profile; you ought to be able to see daylight under the toes and heels.

Virginia: I have traded my Asics Gels for a pair of Rykas. My business partner (and exercise fanatic), Cathy, says they are designed especially for the female foot. I don't know about that, but they feel great and don't slip on my heels. I also wear New Balance shoes that feel great, too. The trick is to find a certified podiatrist to fit the shoes to your feet.

June and Barbara: Then you agree with the experts who say that comfort is all. We advise people to go to a sports shoe shop, where the salespeople are often fanatical walkers or runners themselves and may know more and care more than the department store shoe salesperson. You should insist on a choice of several different brands, and then try each on and walk around a bit—even go outdoors and try them on the sidewalk—until you can decide on the most comfortable. Above all, do not settle for anything but your own size (some salespeople will try to peddle what they have in stock, even if it's a half-size too short or long or narrower or wider than you require). You should have a thumb's width between the end of your toe and the end of the shoe. And a word to women: don't worry about looks. These are not things of beauty, but sports shoes are in style now all over America, so just change your thinking about what is attractive on your feet.

What are these ideally comfortable and well-fitting walking or running shoes going to cost? More than you'll want to pay for a pair for yourself (especially if you're a woman), but about what you would be willing to pay for a pair for your kid: $60 to $90 is not outrageous. The bad news is that when you get into walking twenty or so miles a week, you'll need to toss out the old and bring in the new every six months. As one sports shoe expert told us, you wouldn't want to drive around on worn-out tires with no tread. It's just as bad to walk around on worn-out shoes with no tread. One little money-saving tip is that sometimes you can pick up the earlier model of a newly redesigned shoe at a lesser cost than the latest version. New models come on the market so frequently that the earlier one is usually just as good structurally as the latest edition.

In addition to sport shoes, most comfortable brands of casual shoes, such as those made by Monroe, Rockport, and Ecco, can be used for walking, and they're particularly appropriate for city walking. In New York, the women have worked out a good compromise. They wear sport shoes—usually militantly and grubbily white ones to walk to work—and, once they reach the office, they change into their corporate, go-to-meeting types.

Now for the socks. Seven or eight dollars a pair will buy you socks that will help prevent blisters and/or give you extra padding on the ball of the foot where you might have pain if your fat pad has grown thin over the years or if you tend to build up calluses. As verified by a study in *Diabetes Medicine*, this extra padding may also prevent diabetic foot problems by reducing the pressure on the vulnerable parts of the foot.

The brands of special socks for athletes and people with diabetes have so proliferated of late that it has become rather confusing to figure out which one is best for any individual. For the mail-order companies, you should call and ask questions, explaining your special needs in socks and asking if they have something to meet these requirements. Sources of socks appropriate for people with diabetes are available from Medicool, which describes and advertises its selection of Diasox, Silver Knit socks, TheraSocks, European Comfort socks, Care Sox, and DuraSox in the back of *Diabetes Forecast* magazine (Medicool.com; 1-800-433-2469). Other purveyors of socks for the legendary "diabetic foot" are Theraware, makers of Theraware and SmartKnit seamless socks (theraware.com; 1-866-848-9327), WrightSock.com; (1-800-654-7191), the makers of Anti-Blister and Performance Sport Socks, and Double Lay-R seamfree socks and CoolMax Blister Free socks, (doublelayer.com; 1-800-229-6691).

Virginia: I'd like to add that when buying your shoes, you should wear your padded socks. And I like stores whose salespeople know how to fit you the old-fashioned way. Remember when you were a kid, the salesperson would feel the shoe and tell you whether or not it fit? If you have "at risk" feet, you have diminished sensation and you can't trust your feet to tell you how well the shoe fits. It's not worth saving a few dollars at a discount self-service shoe store and losing a foot.

Now how about telling us how walking becomes an aerobic exercise in the sense that it strengthens the heart and helps control blood pressure?

June and Barbara: You have to walk fast enough to increase your heart rate (number of beats per minute) to at least 65 percent of its maximum rate. That means you have to walk a mile in about seventeen minutes. The standard way of figuring your maximum heart rate is easy: subtract your age from the number 220. For instance, if you're fifty-five, the formula is $220 - 55 = 165$ beats per minute. (You definitely don't want to reach that rate during exercise.) Then take 65 percent of 165 and you get 107 beats per minute. That's your "target rate," but most of you will have to consider your age and physical condition and approach that target slowly. Also, remember Covert Bailey's caution that this formula may not apply to you individually, so you might want to check with your doctor.

To monitor your pulse, check it before, during, and after exercise. Using your fingertips, find your pulse at your wrist (inside) or at the carotid artery underneath your jawbone at the left side of your neck. Count for ten seconds and multiply by six to get your heartbeats per minute. (Our guru Covert Bailey prefers that you count for six seconds and multiply by ten; this does make multiplying easier, but it's harder to count for exactly six seconds because it's such a short time.)

The goal is to keep your heart rate at its target of 60 percent for about twenty to thirty minutes at a time. Only a sustained, uninterrupted effort for this amount of time can condition your heart. This kind of continuous, rhythmical exercise that uses the muscles of the lower body is what's called aerobic exercise. Walking, of course, is only one of many such exercises. You can choose from bicycling, swimming, jogging, aerobic dancing, roller-skating, jumping rope, and others.

Virginia: I get the picture, and I know you start out slowly, with your doctor's approval, if you haven't been doing much of anything in the exercise line. As far as diabetes is concerned, I have to recommend also that you not only monitor your heart rate, but you also monitor your blood sugar if you take pills or insulin, especially insulin. Your blood sugar should be at least 150 before you start your exercise session. If it's less, eat a snack before starting. If it's over 250, there's another factor to consider. There may not be adequate insulin on board to handle the increased demand for fuel that will occur with exercise, and your blood sugar will go up even higher.

In helping patients set up an exercise program, I always explain that they should do their exercise for at least twenty to thirty minutes at a time at least three or four times a week. It should be done at a level that feels somewhat difficult, but not so strenuous that you feel out of breath. And above all, don't exceed your target heart range.

Strength Training

June and Barbara: We hate to remind you that aerobic activity is not the end of the exercise program anymore. All the experts claim now, and we certainly go along with them, that aerobics alone are not enough. You must also do some strength training.

Virginia: You mean pumping iron? Who wants big biceps and show-off muscles? I certainly don't want to look like Popeye, and not many of my patients do, either.

June and Barbara: Don't get us wrong. Neither do we. What is being advocated for health benefits has nothing to do with professional body building. Strength training is done by lifting handheld weights or using weight machines like Nautilus. It's been shown that this kind of training retards the aging process—and you can't knock that. It can make a ninety-year-old as strong as a fifty-year-old. But the biggest news is that it improves insulin sensitivity, and that should make it especially popular with all type 2s who take insulin.

Virginia: Come to think of it, strength training has another great advantage: it improves the body's proportion of muscle to fat, and this really counts from a health standpoint. If your body has a high percentage of fat, it does not require as many calories to preserve that fat. The result is that when you eat extra calories, the body stores them with all that other fat. This is not good news unless you're preparing for a famine. By converting fat to muscle you can change your metabolism so that you burn more calories, which of course helps solve weight problems. This is the secret behind the exercise program Curves. You move around a circuit, spending only thirty seconds on a machine (so little time you can't hurt yourself) and then move to a low-impact board where you walk or jog and then to a different muscle-building machine.

June and Barbara: That's why some health professionals think recommended weight should be determined by measuring the proportion of fat and lean tissue. They don't consider the old height-weight tables to be good guides. We admit that if we followed what's considered normal weight on those tables, we'd be total tubs. But many people feel the federal government's new standard for healthy weight (established in 1998 by the National Institutes of Health [NIH]) has gone too far the other way. This defines anyone with a BMI (body mass index)—a formula used to estimate body fat—of more than 25 as overweight. The definition of obese is a BMI greater than 30. According to these definitions, 55 percent of adult Americans would be considered overweight.

Dr. Xavier Pi-Sunyer, who heads the NIH task force, was quoted in *The Wall Street Journal* as conceding that "the scientific literature doesn't prove conclusively that people with BMIs over 25 will have a shorter life span—unless they have another condition *such as diabetes.*" (Italics are ours.) He also said that the literature doesn't show that people who are overweight according to the new standards are at increased risk of developing health problems, *such as diabetes* and high blood pressure. (Again, the italics are ours.)

This is likely to turn into one of those extended health wrangles until a new controversy comes along to take its place. In the meantime, if you want to check yourself out against this new standard, here's how you do it. (This will make a great parlor game at your next social gathering.) You divide your body weight in kilograms by your height in meters squared. This is tough for Americans, since we don't know our dimensions in the metric system, so you can also just multiply your weight in pounds by 703, and then divide the result by your height in inches. Then divide that result by your height a second time.

$$BMI = \frac{weight\ in\ kilograms\ (total\ pounds \div 2.2)}{height\ in\ meters^2\ (total\ inches\ x\ 2.5 \div 100)}$$

If you don't like how this turns out, you can spend some time and money by getting yourself weighed underwater in a hydrostatic weighing tank. Since fat floats and muscle sinks, the heavier you are underwater, the better. (It's the opposite of the situation on land.) But in your heart of hearts, you probably already know if you're overweight or obese and should do something about it. Women, however, have a tendency to think of themselves as overweight ("I've just got to lose ten pounds!") when they're not, and men have a tendency to think they're not overweight ("I'm just husky") when they are. This test, which is the most accurate, could help people toward a more realistic assessment than working from a chart.

Virginia: Is the above information still valid? There is now lots of data about increased weight increasing risks for diabetes and cardiovascular problems. You can Google BMI and get a BMI calculator to get an exact BMI. I finally hit the other side of 25.

Okay, let's get back to muscle building. How do you get going on it, and how do you learn how to do it?

June and Barbara: It's not as hard as you may think. You don't even have to grunt. In fact, you shouldn't exert yourself that much. And you only have to do it about twice a week. We usually alternate it with our walking exercise, as you don't want to do strength training two days in a row. Your muscles like to rest.

Virginia: If I don't have a gym near where I live, does that mean I can't do muscle strengthening?

June and Barbara: No, it just means you do it at home using free weights. The main problem with that is, unless your diabetes center has an exercise therapist on staff, you'll have to find one to visit or you'll have to buy one of the better books on weight lifting. Two of these are *Designing Resistance Training Programs* by S. J. Fleck and W. J. Kraemer (Champaign, Ill.: Human Kinetics Books, 1987); and *Lift Your Way to Youthful Fitness* by Terry Todd and Jan Todd (Boston: Little, Brown, 1985).

We're lucky because there are plenty of gyms in Southern California where people can get an excellent workout in a short time. There's something motivating about a gym. A Personal Health column of the *Los Angeles Times* about sticking with exercise revealed that women need social support to adopt and maintain an exercise program, while men are motivated by a favorable environment. In a gym you do fraternize with the other exercisers and the environment is more than favorable, because you can't do anything but exercise while you're there. And we find it fun to learn to use the fancy new fitness machines. The gym we used to go to has Nautilus and Cybex equipment. The latter is easy to set, smooth to use, and makes you feel like a real pro.

When you join a gym, you usually get at least one complimentary lesson with a trainer who designs a program just for you. But you have to watch out when signing on, as gyms are now a big business and a very competitive one, and some firms have indulged in fraudulent activities, like signing up hundreds of people and then going out of business or charging excessive start-up fees with the hope that you'll sign on and then drop out within a few months. All have aggressive sales staffs to push you into signing a contract. So beware; you've been warned.

Virginia: Can you give us a brief glimpse of what you actually do during a workout? Some people have never been inside a gym. And are there any cautions for persons with diabetes?

June and Barbara: You're supposed to work at least eight or ten different muscle groups and do one set of each exercise. A set is ten to twelve repetitions ("reps"). For instance, we used to do abdominal, back extension, arm curl, rowing, chest press, lateral pulldown, lateral rise, leg extension, leg curl, and hip adduction. (Those terms are probably mysterious to you, because you have to see the machines to know what they mean.) The load you set the machine for (in five- or ten- pound increments) has to be light enough so that you can lift it at least eight times before your muscles fatigue. If you can lift it more than fifteen times, it's too light. After you've found the appropriate load, work up to about thirty repetitions and then go on to the next heavier weight.

Virginia: How do you keep from injuring yourself? I've known people who strained muscles in gyms.

June and Barbara: Experts William Evans, chief of the human physiology laboratory at the Human Nutrition Research Center on Aging at Tufts University, and Michael Preuss, fitness director at Cooper Aerobics Center in Dallas, give these cautions:

- Lift slowly, avoiding jerky or "explosive" movements. Lifting a weight should take two or three seconds; lowering it should take about the same amount of time.

- Let a trainer in the health club demonstrate proper breathing technique.
- Ask your doctor's advice or get an examination before beginning, especially if you're older or have diabetes or high blood pressure.
- Don't go overboard. An every-other-day program is best.

We would alter that last caution to once or twice a week. And if you have proliferative diabetic retinopathy (a disease of the retina), weight training is a great risk. In fact, get permission from your ophthalmologist if you have even moderate retinopathy. Also talk to your doctor if you have chronic hypertension.

Virginia: I think we all need a rest now. Do you have any final words about exercise?

June and Barbara: We have a final story about weight lifting that we know you'd like to hear.

We read an article in the May 1992 *Diabetes Forecast* that profiled Ron Gillembardo of Las Vegas. Ron was diagnosed with type 2 diabetes in 1982, when he was thirty-eight years old. His blood sugar was 500, and he tipped the scales at 360 pounds. He started working out with weights, and he just happened to excel at it. In less than two years, he lost nearly one hundred pounds, and he got off insulin and onto pills. He kept working out with weights two hours a day, five days a week.

In 1989, Ron began power lifting in competitions. He won almost every competition he entered and became the world record holder in the 710-pound lift. At the age of forty-three he qualified for the 1992 Olympic Games in Barcelona. He is the oldest weight lifter ever to compete in the Olympics.

Now doesn't that make all of you want to get out there and see what kind of prizes you can win with exercise? The best prize, of course, will be your wonderful diabetes control and your new self-esteem.

Transition Time

Now as we pass from one major realm of diabetes control, exercise, to the other major realm, diet, we have the perfect crossover in Virginia's personal true and inspiring tale of weight loss and fitness gain. . . .

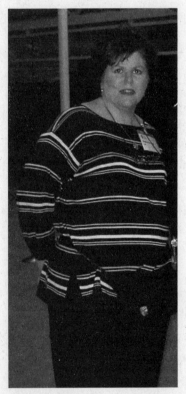

Virginia before

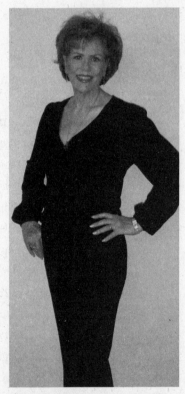

Virginia after

MY EPIPHANY AT THE DALLAS/FORT WORTH AIRPORT

I had one of those life-changing spiritual epiphanies at this most unlikely of places. Trying to get from one gate to the other really fast so I wouldn't miss my connection, I was moving as fast as I could, despite having pain in one leg and feeling really out of breath. As I rushed up to the gate at the last possible minute, a woman around my age (and size) came up to the gate on one of those electric scooters.

Boarding the plane and getting settled into a seat that seemed to be getting smaller and smaller, I was thinking about the lady with the scooter and how I would rather stay home than use a scooter to travel and how that would negatively affect my life. I thought about how much I love the work that I do and that traveling around the country (and the world) and talking about living healthy with diabetes is very important to me. It is more than a job. It is a mission. I realized that if I wanted to continue to do this work I was going to have to be able to travel, and to do so you have to be in pretty good shape. I made up my mind right then and there that I was going to lose weight and get into better shape, so I could be strong enough to walk fast for decent distances and lift my rolling suitcase over my head and put it into the overhead compartment without help. This was January 2003. The "before" picture was taken two years earlier on September 10, 2001, when I was in Scotland at the European Association for the Study of Diabetes (EASD) meeting. I use it as my before picture because in those days I was pretty good at avoiding cameras, but trust me, I was actually about five pounds heavier in January 2003.

So how did I do it? How did I make these monumental—and monumentally necessary—changes? I began slowly by choosing to put only half of whatever food I was selecting on my plate. I discovered that by cutting back (and telling myself I could have more later if I wanted) that usually I was more than satisfied and would not go back for more. In fact, they have done studies on portion sizes, and the larger the portion in front of you, the more you will eat. (This is how the United States has become "supersized.")

The other thing I did was look for opportunities to exercise. My friend Debbie and I would make it a point to go to the farmers' market on Saturday mornings and always walked the entire area (while buying some good veggies). With all this diet and exercise focus, by October 2003 I had lost about eight or ten pounds.

Then, two beneficial things happened. I got into a clinical trial for Symlin (more about that drug later) and joined Curves. It promotes itself as "a gym where women change their lives thirty minutes at a time." Unlike a lot of advertising, this turned out to be true. If you go there only three times a week at thirty minutes a whack, you can make a big change in yourself.

Over the next year and a half I lost another eighteen pounds, but I also got a lot stronger. In fact, that is one of the things I really like about Curves; after about the first two weeks, I felt amazingly stronger without causing any injuries. And I began to see a real difference; every ten to fifteen pounds is a dress size. I was thrilled with this level of weight loss and feeling much better when Byetta came on the market and wow!

At this point I am down to about 110 units of insulin a day on my pump (down from 150–160) thanks to my weight loss and Byetta. Since I understand how it works (more later about that), I know that I need to greatly decrease my mealtime insulin (Humalog in my pump), so I cut my usual meal bolus on the pump by half. I could not believe the effect. First, I was soooo not hungry (I could hardly eat one-quarter of my usual portions), and second, my after-meal blood glucose was staying in the normal range . . . like

100–120! I was amazed . . . I had a little nausea for the first three injections but that went away. I just told myself, "Hey, you are not pregnant and you're not eating. It's all good." That's when my weight loss really took off, and within a few months I no longer needed mealtime insulin. After two years, I had lost seventy pounds and am now taking glipizide 10 at bedtime and Byetta twice a day. No insulin. In fairness, Byetta is approved to be used in combination with oral agents, not insulin. Using it in combination with insulin is considered "off label" use, but I figure we are all on insulin, one way or the other. We make it or we take it. I still go to Curves to maintain my weight loss because I am convinced that exercise doesn't take weight off unless you are doing something really strenuous for a few hours a day. After five years I have lost 100 pounds! I am maintaining a BMI of 22 in the normal range. The body mass index is a way to put the ratio of your height and weight into one number. As you can imagine, knowing only your weight doesn't tell you whether you are at a good weight or not. It depends on how tall you are . . . for many years I was simply under tall. You can Google BMI and find lots of calculators, and usually your doctor or diabetes educator will have a chart somewhere in their office. If your BMI is between 25 and 29, you are considered overweight and, if over 30, obese. They have several classifications of obese, but I simplified it: if you are over 40, we consider your weight to be "overbese."

My A1C? Always good, around 5.9 or 6, now 4.9 or 5. And I feel "normal," which is about ten times better than "good."

Designing a Weight-Loss Program with Byetta

Virginia: I recently had a great time on a six month diabetes education tour for Byetta with Delta Burke of *Designing Women* fame. Delta has always been a hero to me, since like so many of us she has struggled with her weight, and she has had to struggle in public. It was very interesting being in a booth with her answering questions about Byetta and diabetes and listening to the questions people ask. Most commonly, people wanted to know how she lost so much weight (sixty-five pounds). She reminds them that it took many years. (I can relate to that. It took me more than four years to lose seventy-two pounds). The most significant thing that she tells people: "I changed my mind about my weight . . . instead of constantly beating myself up for being fat and not losing weight, I began to appreciate myself for not *gaining* weight. I would give myself credit for maintaining my weight and I stopped being so hard on myself all the time." In the last two years she lost twenty pounds on Byetta. I, myself, have dropped seventy pounds since I started on Byetta and a total of 100 pounds in more than five years.

June and Barbara: Since Byetta is still fairly new on the diabetes scene, could you fill us in on what it is and what it does?

Virginia: First off, Byetta is an incretin. That is to say, it belongs to a group of "gut hormones" that help with metabolism. These increcretins have only been understood for the last twenty years. The most well understood one is GLP-1. I call it the "helper hormone." Your body starts making this in the intestines as soon as you begin eating. It helps your body with a number of important functions so you can have a normal after-meal blood sugar.

Byetta works by kicking up the beta cells in the pancreas to make insulin correctly. All of us with diabetes have lost our first-phase insulin squirt. This is very important, as it helps tell the liver to quit making so much glucose because there is food on its way.

It tells the liver to settle down. This is significant because a lot of folks have really high glucose levels after meals and they can't understand why eating a small meal with very few carbohydrates can cause such high postprandial (after-meal) glucose levels. By correcting the action of the "alpha cells" in the pancreas (they make glucagon and tell your liver to make extra glucose) the liver quits making so much glucose after the meal and that helps keep your blood sugars normal.

It slows the emptying of the stomach. Most of us folks with diabetes have fast emptying of our stomachs, therefore putting too much glucose into the bloodstream right after eating. It impacts hunger centers in the brain to tell you when to stop eating.

Now the problem is that folks with type 2 diabetes are deficient in that helpful GLP-1 hormone. Even when they're in the prediabetes state, people can start losing their GLP-1. We could replace it now that we know how to make replicas of hormones (that's how we make "human" insulin), but unfortunately we make an enzyme that degrades the hormone within two minutes of making it. This hormone is called DPP-4.

So we have two possible ways to solve this problem. One of these is to develop an "analog" (a close representation of the original) to GLP-1, but one that would be resistant to the effects of DPP-4. This brings us back to Byetta.

Byetta is a medication that was identified several years ago when a scientist noticed a substance in the saliva of the Gila (pronounced HEEL-A) monster—yes that is a poisonous lizard that lives in Arizona. This has all the action of human GLP-1, but it is *slightly* different than human GLP-1 in that it is resistant to DPP-4 and it lasts six to ten hours.

The other way to solve the problem would be to block the DPP-4 enzyme. We have lots of medications that are enzyme blockers, such as the main group of blood pressure medications, ACE inhibitors (ACE stands for angiotensin converting enzyme). The problem is that we are already GLP-1 deficient, so making it last longer only helps a little.

So to sum it up, here is the good and bad news on the two possible solutions:

Byetta (exenatide) is taken by injection—I guess some would call that bad news—before the two largest meals of the day, but it also comes in a pen that is very easy to use. The good news is most people lose weight and their average A1C reduction can range anywhere from 1 percent to 2 percent. Even better, it makes you feel really full so you don't even want to overeat. For the first time in my life, I was able to eat less than half my plate and push it away.

Januvia (sitagliptin) is an oral pill, which most people prefer—although they will often choose the Byetta when they realize that they will get weight loss with Byetta versus weight neutral effect (stays the same) from Januvia. Also, in clinical trials, Januvia seems to lower A1C about 0.5 percent to 1 percent from baseline glucose.

In my clinical practice, I will often use Januvia with good success on folks who are early into diabetes and have only a modest A1C elevation (just a little over 7). If the patient is seriously interested in weight loss and needs more A1C reduction, they will often choose Byetta. One thing I have to warn these people is that few of them will have the weight-loss success that I have had in the last few years. I have lost more than seventy-two pounds in over four years, but I have been working on it constantly by going to Curves consistently and trying to stay focused on portion size and choosing healthier foods.

In my Byetta patients, the average weight loss is ten to twelve pounds. One thing that I have found helps is to take it an hour before eating to enhance the appetite-reducing effect. I'm really looking forward to the next generation of Byetta coming in about two years—it will only require a once-a-week injection. In early studies it seems to have an even better effect on glucose and weight loss. But the most exciting thing about these new meds is that they appear to restore beta cell function and mass. In the rats they increased the amount of beta cells making insulin in the pancreas. So conceivably, if you could start on one of these meds while in the prediabetes state, you might prevent diabetes altogether. That would be the best news of all.

4

Food, Diet, Nutrition

The "Only More So" Disease

PEOPLE WITH DIABETES ARE NOT THAT DIFFERENT FROM the rest of the population. When you come right down to it, for optimum health, a person with type 2 diabetes needs to do what anyone else should do—only more so. Everybody needs to be on an exercise program; so does the person with diabetes—only more so. All inhabitants of the modern world need to learn how to handle personal and work and societal stresses; so does the person with diabetes—only more so.

Never does the "only more so" factor apply more strongly than in the area of diet. Everyone needs to follow a healthy diet, but people with diabetes need to follow one that is even more healthy than the average person's. But the big question these days is, what is a healthy diet? Reports issued by the U.S. Surgeon General,

National Institutes of Health, American Heart Association, American Dietetic Association, American Medical Association, as well as battalions of medical and dietary experts (and self-proclaimed experts) all tell us the right diet to follow. But they point in so many different—and constantly changing—directions that we often don't know which way to go. In our erstwhile publication, *The Diabetic Reader,* we included a regular column called The Fickle Finger of Food Facts. In each issue we reported the new pronouncements that negated the previous ones: coffee, which was a bad thing one year, is declared harmless the next; we were told to cut back drastically on salt for a period, and then suddenly we were warned that many people weren't getting enough salt, causing them to have a sodium deficiency; at the urging of Linus Pauling and others we loaded up on vitamin C for cold prevention and antioxidant benefits, then came an assertion that vitamin C has prooxidant as well as antioxidant effects, and therefore could cause genetic damage if taken in large doses; one month, soybeans and tofu are supposed to cure everything that ails you, the next month they're implicated in Alzheimer's disease. Everybody is totally confused—and people with diabetes are even more so.

We're going to do our best to alleviate some of the diabetes dietary confusion, but it won't be easy. Just as in Supreme Court decisions, we have a majority opinion and a minority opinion. The conservative majority says that the best diet for type 2s is high in complex carbohydrates and fiber and low in fat. The so-called radical minority believes that a low-carbohydrate diet with more protein, and therefore fat, is the answer. Between the three of us we'll try just like attorneys to defend both positions and explain some of the secondary—but still important—dietary considerations along the way. When you discover the diet or, more likely, dietary variations that work best for you, you'll find that before long you'll look and feel as healthy, vital, and vibrant as your contemporaries without diabetes.

—*June and Barbara*

Swimming in the Conservative Mainstream: The Low-Fat, High-Carbohydrate, High-Fiber Diet

June and Barbara: When people are diagnosed with type 2 diabetes, they're usually told that with a little bit of luck they can probably control their blood sugar level simply by changing their diet and adding regular exercise. This is a comforting thought, compared with taking blood sugar–lowering pills or injections of insulin, but is it true?

Virginia: Yes, in many cases type 2 diabetes can be managed with diet and weight loss. Statistics tell us that among people with type 2 diabetes, 40 percent control their diabetes with pills, and about 35 percent with insulin. This means that less than 25 percent are controlling blood sugar with diet and exercise alone—usually that's a code for "doing nothing," because too often the person with type 2 has not been referred to a nutritionist or an exercise program. Does this mean that two-thirds of all type 2s are bad people who don't follow a proper diet? No, these statistics probably reflect the evolution of the disease.

Initially, the disease is manifested primarily in insulin resistance and is amenable to treatment with diet and exercise. As the insulin deficiency becomes more severe, the need for oral agents and sometimes with a bit of insulin increases. Eventually, when the insulin deficiency and excessive liver glucose production outstrip the pills' ability to control blood sugars, insulin becomes essential.

When I was at the Presbyterian Diabetes Center, we suggested what we call the Fast Fast to help many people get their blood sugars into control quickly, or to get off medications if they're already using them. (**Note:** If you decide you want to try a Fast Fast, be sure to consult with your doctor. They like to be in on such things.)

The Fast Fast is not really a fast. It's a fast from carbohydrates only. (All foods are composed of various combinations of carbohydrate, protein, and fat; carbohydrates are sugars and starches, and they usually account for about 50 percent of what we eat.) On the Fast Fast you can eat as much salad with low-fat dressing as you want. You eat at least one small meat serving a day, baked, broiled, or boiled, and all the sugar-free gelatin you can stand, any color. You can also have all the sugar-free sodas, coffee, and tea you want, but on top of that you should be sure to drink at least eight large glasses of water a day.

The "Fast Fast"

June and Barbara: How do most people feel while on the Fast Fast?

Virginia: They usually don't feel bad at all. What happens is that they get a headache the first day and then they're not even hungry after that.

We always have people on the Fast Fast test their blood sugar at least twice a day, because blood sugars can drop precipitously. People on insulin or pills will need a health professional to coach them so they know how to decrease their medication in anticipation of the lowering blood sugars. Otherwise they might get too low and run out and attack a doughnut shop or something. To get off the pills or insulin and achieve the goal glucose level takes three to five days. Then you start adding carbohydrates . . . slowly. First add low-carbohydrate green vegetables such as green beans, broccoli, and spinach. Even though they're green, peas are almost pure starch, so don't add them yet. Avocados are high in fat, so don't add them. Next try adding toast for breakfast, then maybe a potato at dinner. In other words, gradually add one carbohydrate at a time to see the effect on your blood sugar.

Let me tell you about Mary Jane, a nurse who works nights and has had type 2 diabetes for eight or ten years. She was one of the students in a nursing course I was teaching for the University of Phoenix in Albuquerque. She introduced herself, rather proudly, as a noncompliant person with diabetes. (At the time, she was unaware of what I did for a living.) She was a typical picture of a person with diabetes who had been blamed for her disease for so long that she pinned the "noncompliant" label on herself before anyone else had a chance. She was seventy-five pounds overweight and taking large amounts of insulin, but still her blood glucose levels usually ran from 200 to 400. She felt bad all the time, and was helpless to stop her cycle of overeating and poor control. Worst of all, she believed her problems were all her own fault.

After we had known each other for a few weeks, Mary Jane came up to me after class and described how she would wake up with low blood sugar every afternoon and eat the house down for the rest of the evening. Then she'd go to work at 10:30 p.m. and feel awful. (Her insulin regimen was the same as if she had been on a day schedule.) I asked her to let me know when she was ready to get off insulin, and I would help her.

She waited a few weeks before she brought up the subject. I told her how to do the Fast Fast, lowering her insulin as her blood glucose levels came down. (Since she was a nurse, she could be trusted to handle this on her own.) She called me on the weekend to complain that she felt awful. She wasn't used to having blood glucose levels in the normal range; of course, she felt entirely different from when she was 200 to 300 all the time. But even though she felt bad, boy, was she excited and happy because she was off insulin.

She had an appointment with her doctor for that next week. I told her to ask him for a prescription for an oral hypoglycemic agent so that she would have a safety net if her blood glucose levels started going up a little as she gradually added back carbohydrate food. We also spent a great deal of time talking about how to eat light, low-fat meals and about starting to exercise.

Her doctor was shocked that she was off insulin and that her fasting blood glucose was down to 185. (She would get lower than that throughout the day, but that pesky liver would pop it up during the night, and that's why she needed the pills.) The doctor suggested she go back on insulin, and Mary Jane rightly replied, "Remember what my blood glucose level was when I was on insulin?" On top of that, she was now twelve pounds lighter. By taking Diabeta pills (she calls them Diabetter) and getting back on carbohydrates, she is keeping her blood glucose levels between 100 and 200 and has lost a total of thirty-five pounds. She's exercising at least three hours a week and is feeling better than she has in years.

June and Barbara: The Fast Fast sounds like a miracle cure, but Mary Jane had had diabetes for eight or ten years. Does the Fast Fast work equally well for those newly diagnosed with diabetes?

Virginia: Yes, in fact, better. I have another success story for you that proves it. I met Nick in the hospital. His doctor had hospitalized him as a newly diagnosed person with diabetes, although most endocrinologists, instead of putting patients in the hospital, refer them to diabetes educator nurses and dietitians to do their initial training and glucose control as outpatients. Nick, a good-looking though chubby Hispanic guy about thirty-five years old, is a computer programmer who leads a pretty sedentary life. He had gone to the doctor with symptoms of excess urination, excess thirst, and generally feeling awful. He suspected diabetes, because most of the people in his family over the age of sixty had the disease. He had not lost large amounts of weight during this period of illness. In fact, he was about fifty pounds overweight.

The doctor had him on 70/30 insulin (NPH and regular premixed in a vial) and wanted him to get a blood glucose testing meter. I was to teach him how to use the meter. His blood sugars were still moderately high, in the 200s. I told him that it would be useful for him to be on insulin, because otherwise in those days his health insurance would not pay for a meter. But I promised him that we could get him off insulin pronto, whenever he was ready. He looked at me as if I were crazy. I think the doctor must have told him I was crazy, because we didn't see him again for a few months.

He finally decided to come to our eight-week course. He was still on insulin, but his dose was lower. He had lost about ten pounds because his wife was following the diet guidelines given to them in the hospital. When he showed up in class, he asked me about getting off insulin. I said, "Sure, Nick, whenever you're ready." I knew it wouldn't be difficult, because he was on so little insulin—about 16 units in the morning and 10 at night. If he really needed insulin, it would have taken a lot more than that for a guy weighing more than two hundred pounds. Besides, when you're young and brand new to diabetes, the Fast Fast works especially well.

He started on the Fast Fast and in a few days was normoglycemic (another word for euglycemic) and off insulin.

June and Barbara: We're happy to hear you talk about people getting off insulin. There's a terrible rumor going around that once you start taking insulin you have to take it forever. One type 2 woman, who had always been controlled with diet and exercise, wrote to us of a terrifying experience for her. She had been hospitalized for surgery and the stress caused her blood sugars to go up. When her doctors told her they were going to give her some insulin to bring it down, she fainted dead away. That was because she thought she was going to be on insulin for the rest of her life. After her recovery, her blood sugar went back down, and she could again control her diabetes without insulin. "But," she complained, "why did I have to go through that when it wasn't necessary? Why didn't someone explain to me that this was just a temporary thing?" Why indeed? Let's hear it for letting the patient know what's going on! But how about Nick? Is he still off insulin?

Virginia: Yes, he's continued to keep his blood glucose in control with diet and exercise. He has a nice blood glucose meter to keep track of it, thanks to his health insurance. If Nick can keep losing weight, he'll probably be able to control his diabetes for many years with diet and exercise. This is not to say that the disease was solely caused by his diet, his obesity, or his sedentary lifestyle. Those factors were certainly not in his favor, but we know lots of guys just like Nick—overweight, sedentary lifestyle—who don't have diabetes. Remember, type 2 diabetes is a genetic disease, not a character flaw.

Low-Fat Lifestyle

June and Barbara: Many people newly diagnosed with diabetes are sent by their doctors to a dietitian. In our opinion, this is definitely the way to go. People think the dietitian will tell them to get off sugar forever, but instead the talk is mostly about fat. We also noticed that at the Diabetes Network you have a teaching manual that recommends a low-fat lifestyle. Why is fat such a big deal for people with type 2 diabetes?

Virginia: You're right in noticing that fat is a big deal. People with type 2 diabetes have a metabolic defect that causes their bodies to prefer fat over glucose as a fuel source. People without diabetes normally use glucose as their fuel of preference. The glucose is shuttled into the muscle cells via the cells' receptors, thanks to insulin "opening the door." Glucose is used strictly as fuel; fat goes into storage.

Now let's say you're a type 2 and your muscle cell receptors don't work so well. They can't make use of the insulin to get the glucose into the cell. One thing Mother Nature did for us as a safety valve was to give us the ability to use fatty acids as well as glucose for fuel. So when they can't get to the glucose, your muscles can use fatty acids as their fuel to keep going.

When you eat a meal with 50 percent of the calories from fat, here come the two fuels, fat and glucose, floating down the bloodstream to meet your muscles. The muscles would actually prefer the glucose, but what will they do if they can't get the glucose in? They grab the fat and use it as their fuel and leave the glucose floating around. High-fat diets have been shown to increase insulin resistance. That's why you end up with high blood sugar after a high-fat meal; it has a glucose-sparing effect.

This is not the way it works in people who don't have diabetes. In a normal person, fat goes straight into storage and doesn't raise the blood sugar. Fat is not sugar. It doesn't even convert to blood sugar except under extreme circumstances.

But the person with type 2 diabetes has high blood sugar because his or her body used the fat for fuel instead of the glucose; the insulin level is high as well because the pancreas is making more insulin to deal with the high blood sugar. Now the insulin is going to store the glucose as fat. So into storage it goes, and the type 2 gains more weight.

A recent article in *Obesity Journal* (before I lost all that weight, I was asked to be the centerfold but declined) looked at a large number of people with and without diabetes and measured their body fat levels and then tracked their eating habits over a long period of time. The researchers noted two things: one, thin people and fat people eat about the same amount of calories (this was already a well-known fact); and two, thin people eat less than 30 percent of their calories as fat, and fat people eat more than 30 percent of their calories as fat. This is the big difference.

So can we cut our fat consumption to 10, 20, or 25 percent of our calories and lose weight? The jury is still out on this, but for some people, it is certainly looking like the way to go. For the person with diabetes, this is neither as easy nor as difficult as it sounds. If you cut the fat, you have to add carbohydrates in order to have enough calories. To prevent the high-carbohydrate diet from raising your blood glucose levels, you have to be careful to add lots of fiber. If in combination with a low-fat and high-fiber diet you also get plenty of exercise, you'll not only lose weight, but you'll be the healthiest you could ever be. This is what we call the "low-fat lifestyle," and if it's beginning to sound familiar, it should. It is the recommendation for a healthy heart, cancer prevention, and good health in general.

We advise people not to think of this as a diet. People who go on diets also go off diets. We ask our patients to go on a life plan. Eating less than 20 percent to 30 percent fat requires some fundamental changes, but if you give yourself plenty of the carbohydrates that you love and add protein as well, you'll feel great and not get into the deprivation mode, a surefire way to blow your diet.

June and Barbara: Many experts agree that fat, not carbohydrate, is the real enemy. Avoiding fat is the cornerstone of the successful Pritikin weight-loss (and health-gain!) diet and of the Martin Katahn T-Factor diet. It's also basic in Dr. James Anderson's high-carbohydrate, high-fiber, low-fat diet (HCF diet), which allows only 9 percent calories as fat but so improves insulin sensitivity in · people with type 2 diabetes that in one study the diet resulted in 52 percent of overweight type 2s being taken off insulin completely.

Now tell us exactly how you follow a low-fat diet.

Virginia: Get obsessed with fat. Look for it everywhere. Get a calorie and nutrient counter paperback at the bookstore and start looking at every label of every food product you consider buying. To find out how many grams of fat you can have, estimate your total daily calories—for example, 1,600. Now multiply by 30 percent to find out how many calories of fat you can have. This would be 480. Now divide those calories by 9 to determine the grams of fat you can have (each gram of fat has 9 calories). The answer is 53. (That's 10 or 11 fat exchanges if you use the American Diabetes Association's exchange lists.) Fifty-three grams of fat are plenty to keep you dietarily happy.

Look at breakfast, for example. Skim milk has no fat. (I use 1/2 percent milk to avoid the transparent look of skim, but that's only 1 gram of fat per cup, whereas low-fat milk contains 5 grams a cup.) Cheerios (and many other cereals, hot or cold) are fat free. A banana is fat free. Hey, this is really easy . . . no problem.

Now, how about lunch? You were going to eat macaroni and cheese? Think again. A typical serving (about twice the recommended amount) has 35 grams of fat—two-thirds of your whole day's supply. You really have to watch cheeses. In fact, most cheese recipes are high in fat; you know, a little leftover this and that and cover it with about a cup of grated cheddar and voila, a culinary masterpiece.

So what are some good choices for lunch? Try a baked potato topped with low-fat cottage cheese and chives, which tastes better than sour cream. How about pasta with a tomato and mushroom sauce with no meat? You should keep the pasta down to one cup. If that still leaves you feeling hungry, add a salad with fat-free dressing and a vegetable such as zucchini or green beans. If you want meat, make it skinless chicken, fish, or a very small serving of lean red meat. You'll have to be very careful about eating meat. In many cases, half the calories in a meat serving come from fat. Put another way, the quarter-pound hamburger patty (three ounces cooked) has 10 to 15 grams of fat—and that's without cheese or mayonnaise.

Dinner? Well, you must be getting the idea by now. Just get out that fat gram counter and you'll be safe.

By the way, all fats are not created equal. Some fats are considered to be "good fats," and others are considered "bad fats." The good fats are monounsaturated fats, as opposed to saturated fats. Saturated fats are butter fats and those that come from the fat of meat. Monofats are fats from canola oil, peanut oil, olive oil, and my favorite green vegetable, avocado. These fats may actually increase your HDL (the good cholesterol), so when you do eat some fat, you should choose fats from these sources if possible.

June and Barbara: It's really important to have a fat gram counter and understand clearly where fat lurks in food. A lot of people just don't get it. During the 1992 Republican convention, we heard a radio interview from a Houston barbecue place that was a favorite of then-president Bush since back when he was in the oil business in that city. Bush had stopped by to eat while he was in town for the convention. The interviewer asked the owner of the place what Bush had selected for his meal. She said that he had barbecued beef, barbecued ribs, and hot links with coleslaw. She said that normally he would have had baked beans instead of the coleslaw, but he had told her he was on a low-fat diet. Wowee! The only thing that might possibly have been low-fat in that place were the baked beans—assuming they weren't loaded with bacon or ham.

To keep you from inadvertently living off the fat of the land, we'd like to suggest a few fat gram counters so you can run right out and buy one while you're fired up on the idea. There's a huge choice, but we'll only list the ones you're most likely to find in your local bookstore or on the Internet:

- *CalorieKing Calorie, Fat and Carbohydrate Counter* (also has lots of great restaurant information)
- *The Corinne T. Netzer Fat Gram Counter*
- *The Fat Counter* by Annette Natow and Jo-Ann Heslin
- *The T-Factor 2000 Fat Gram Counter* (Revised and Updated Edition) by Jamie Pope-Cordle and Martin Katahn
- *Vest Pocket Fat Counter* by Susan Podell
- *The Ultimate Calorie, Carb & Fat Gram Counter* by Lea Ann Holzmeister
- *Crazy Plates: Low-Fat Food So Good, You'll Swear It's Bad for You* by Janet Podleski

When you come right down to it, just how easy—or hard—is it for most people to follow such a low-fat diet?

Virginia: Take it from one who's done it: it's not easy to get out there and live in the real world on a really low-fat diet. Temptation is ubiquitous. The first rule of thumb is, if it's fried, forget it! Cheese is a real no-no. This is the most painful part for me. I love cheese! At home I use the fat-free or low-fat cheese slices (Kraft Free, Lite Line, and Alpine Lace are good ones), although they're a little salty for my taste because I also cut down on salt. There are a few dishes that you need a little bit of cheese for, and these nonfat or low-fat varieties do the trick. They even melt nicely.

Another thing I really miss is mayonnaise. There are some good low-fat mayonnaises such as Hellmann's Light, which has half the fat of regular mayo, but even so it has 5 grams of fat per serving. Kraft makes a fat-free mayo, but as far as taste goes—yuck! I have discovered that I can buy some extremely good low-fat dressings. I've found one with Parmesan and garlic (boy, is that good!), and I use that mixed with tuna to make a sandwich. On turkey or chicken sandwiches I use mustard, which is totally fat free.

How are you going to eat a potato without any fat on it? Besides low-fat cottage cheese with chives or green onion, try salsa. It gives the potato a really nice flavor.

Restaurant Dining

June and Barbara: It's one thing when you're at home and in total control of the situation, but how about when you eat out? Eating in a restaurant is the hardest part of any diet—especially a low-fat one. Maybe you could give us a few tips on how you handle that.

Virginia: Well, living in Albuquerque as I do, my favorite food when dining out is our wonderful New Mexican cuisine. A typical local food is enchiladas. They dip a tortilla in oil then in chile (a sauce of red chile, not like Texas chili), put cheese in it and fold it over, then pour green chile over it and add more cheese—plenty of cheese! They also serve a lot of refried beans. The classic way to make refried beans is to start with pinto beans and add a cup or two of lard or bacon drippings.

Fortunately, my favorite restaurant prepares its beans with no fat. They're nothing but cooked pinto beans mashed up. They taste just as good as the refried ones with all the fat—maybe even better, since you feel so virtuous when you eat them. Of course, I don't get the enchiladas. I order off the à la carte menu and pick fat-free dishes. For instance, they have an excellent dish called potatoes Garcia. It's just sliced potatoes cooked down until they're real soft, with cilantro and a touch of green chile added. Boy, are they good! No fat and wonderful flavor. I get a big tortilla and eat the beans and potatoes mixed up with a little green chile. Green chile sauce has little or no fat. You can be selective like this in any restaurant. When you order fish, ask them to grill or broil it and leave off the fat. Skip the sauce, too. Most restaurants are happy to do that for you.

When I go into a restaurant and order a meal that includes a piece of meat that is much larger than I need, I know I'll eat it all if it's on my plate, so I ask my husband to split the entrée with me. We each order our own potato and salad. That way I'll be quite satisfied with a serving of two or three ounces of meat.

June and Barbara: We handle that too-large protein serving in a different way. We each order a full portion but take half of it home in a doggie bag. It's not too hard to resist the temptation to eat all of it if you know the leftovers will save you the trouble of shopping for and fixing a protein course at home the next night.

You can ask for doggie bags even in the best restaurants. We have a friend who is very socially prominent and has gone to the fanciest of private finishing schools. She now works as a volunteer at UCLA giving conversation classes to newly arrived foreign students. They ask her questions about experiences they've had that were confusing or upsetting to them. One Korean girl told our friend she was out to dinner with her boyfriend and at the end of the meal the waiter asked her if she wanted a doggie bag. She said, "I was so frightened! I didn't know what to say or do." Our friend explained what a doggie bag is and assured the student that she should never hesitate to ask for one because everybody does it and it's a perfectly correct thing to do. If she says it's okay, it must be!

Virginia: Another good tip is to ask for the doggie bag at the beginning of the meal. Put half of your meat portion in it, and then you won't be tempted to eat the whole portion on your plate. Most of us have found that we must play lots of little games with ourselves to make our diets work. One trick is to focus on permissible foods. What you can have makes a wonderful life, because you can feel good and you can have health.

June and Barbara: Some people who are genuine fatophobes may want to know if it's okay to eliminate all fat in an individual meal.

Virginia: It's difficult to totally eliminate 100 percent of the fat, although it's not impossible. You'll find, though, that if you eat a fat-free meal it's also probably virtually a protein-free meal and that means you'll get a pretty steep glucose rise after the meal. As I suggested previously, if you're on insulin, you can learn to cover the carbohydrate with your insulin dose. For most people, the formula is one unit of regular insulin (fast-acting) or Humalog for each 10 grams of carbohydrate. You can do that and then do a one-hour after-meal blood sugar reading to determine your own formula for covering food with insulin. Another tip for those still using regular insulin is to take it at least forty-five minutes before eating a high-carb meal so the insulin will peak with the food. (If you are on Humalog, of course, you can take it right before you eat.)

I would like to comment, though, that no one would want to entirely eliminate fat 100 percent of the time because there are some incredibly important vitamins that we get from fat. These are the so-called fat-soluble vitamins A, D, E, and K. Vitamin E is very important for keeping our skin soft and wrinkle free (as if that were possible!). It's also important for healing and we would not want to slow that down. If you eat a normal diet of a little bit of meat here and there, use some olive oil once in a while on a salad, and have some dairy products (skim milk is fortified with vitamin D), you'll be safe on these vitamins. Also, remember that not all fats are "bad" fats.

June and Barbara: Are you saying there is such a thing as "good" fat?

Virginia: Yes, the monounsaturated fats (described on page 157) are good for us. They still have 9 calories per gram but contribute to a healthy heart. I have discovered a margarine called Canola Harvest that tastes really good and is made completely from canola oil.

Binge Eating

June and Barbara: Jane Brody, health columnist for *The New York Times*, wrote a column about a new category of eating disorder, distinct from anorexia or bulimia and far more common than either of these. It's called binge eating disorder and accounts for a large proportion of seriously overweight Americans who repeatedly try to lose weight but fail. You've probably met hundreds of people with diabetes who fit this description. If binge eating disorder is their problem, they indulge in frequent, uncontrolled, and often hours-long eating episodes during which they may devour more than 2,000 calories. Psychologist Richard R. Rubin calls these "search and consume missions." Unlike people with bulimia, they do not attempt to purge their bodies of the excess calories by inducing vomiting or taking laxatives. They simply gain weight.

According to Dr. Robert L. Spitzer, who proposed that this disorder be included in the official manual of psychiatric diagnoses so that insurance would reimburse for its treatment, binge eaters tend to be depressed, anxious, or suffering other psychological disturbances much more than other people with comparable weight problems. Here are the criteria to identify the condition:

- Recurrent episodes of bingeing and the sense that the eating is out of control.
- Episodes occur at least twice a week on average, for six months or longer.
- The behavior causes marked distress.
- Binges involve at least three of these actions: eating much more rapidly than usual; eating to uncomfortable fullness; eating large amounts of food even when not hungry; eating alone out of embarrassment; eating out of feelings of disgust or guilt.

Unfortunately, going on a diet does not solve this problem; in fact, drastic dieting may trigger bingeing behavior. Overeaters Anonymous is a good form of group therapy for bingers. In fact, Dr. Spitzer's study found that 71 percent of participants in Overeaters Anonymous met his diagnostic criteria for binge eating disorder.

From your experience with seriously overweight people who have diabetes, would you say that many of them have this psychological problem? If so, will treating it put them on the road to weight loss?

Virginia: I'm sure that Dr. Spitzer is onto something here. I frequently encounter patients who use the very words, "My eating is out of control." There is one more stimulus he hasn't noted that I feel may be very significant for a type 2. As you proceed down the merry path of type 2 diabetes—highly insulin resistant, taking excessive amounts of insulin to control your blood glucose, but even so, only partially controlling it—your blood glucose goes up incrementally. In other words, you can sort of control your blood glucose, but if it goes up due to a dietary indiscretion—such as if you "accidentally" ate a chocolate bunny for Easter—your body cannot bring it back down and you will stay at the higher level. This is the phenomenon we've called glucose toxicity. It is a condition where your insulin works better at normal range glucoses. It also takes a lot more insulin to conquer a high blood glucose than to maintain a normal range.

June and Barbara: June can certainly verify this. If her blood sugar is in the low 200s, it takes a supplement of only one unit of insulin to return her to normal blood glucose (90–100). But if she gets wildly out of control, say the high 200s or low 300s, it takes two units to get her back down to 200, plus a third unit to get her down to normal. She's lucky enough to be able to get back on track by injecting supplements of insulin, but as you point out, those type 2s who don't take insulin just stay up there.

Virginia: That's why we do the Fast Fast. It brings blood glucose down quickly. You become more sensitive to your own insulin, and if you keep your blood glucose normal for a while, then you can often control it by watching your diet and you'll be less likely to have hunger attacks.

One reason why many type 2s binge is the huge amount of insulin they're getting, especially when their blood glucose is out of control. As a type 2 myself, I can "feel" an insulin rush during and after meals. It feels a little like the insulin reaction (blood glucose going too low) that type 1s get when they overdose on insulin. When I'm getting an insulin surge I feel my lips quiver, but when I look in the mirror they aren't moving. Sometimes I get a little quivery feeling in my chest or neck. This is why many type 2s will tell you that they aren't hungry all day—until they eat something. They get a rush of insulin with the food and that gives them the munchies. Then they proceed to eat all evening long. I'm sure that June can confirm this feeling. When you feel a surge of insulin in your body, it is very difficult not to eat something. I've found that if I can explain this reaction to people, they can live with it—and cope with it—better. For years they've probably been beating themselves up about having no willpower.

Besides these insulin surges that cause overeating, I feel that getting yourself into a "deprivation" mode can trigger the binge disorder; at least it does for me. That's why a diet of 20 percent to 30 percent fat works so well. The fact that you don't limit your serving sizes on the good-for-you foods (like veggies and low-fat protein foods) gives you the strength to avoid the bad stuff. We have a patient with type 2, a woman of thirty-five who has lost thirty pounds in the last four months. One day she told me, "I can live like this forever, because I know I can have what I want when it comes to veggies and low-fat protein foods." I'm confident that she's going to be able to avoid the pitfall of the deprivation mode and binge eating.

Carbohydrates

June and Barbara: In the recommended diets, sugar has always been a no-no, until the recent ADA pronouncements, but starch is okay. Why is this? Aren't they both carbohydrates?

Virginia: As it turns out, there's very little difference. The biochemist calls starch a complex carbohydrate because it is a long chain of glucose molecules, as opposed to simple sugars that are made up of only a few glucose molecules. Dietitian Beverly Spears uses a great visual demonstration for this concept. She has several strings of those great big pop beads babies play with, which she has the patient break apart. Guess what? The long chain breaks apart just as easily as the short chain. This is the reason that the glycemic index studies found that white starches and white sugar are not very different in the effect they have on blood sugar. The glycemic index is a tool to measure the relative effect that different foods have on blood glucose. Different glycemic index studies have shown that white rice, mashed potatoes, and sugar have a similar effect on blood glucose. Does that mean that the person with diabetes should not eat potatoes or white rice? No, what it means is that you shouldn't eat a big bowl of white rice or mashed potatoes for a meal. A study reported in the *Diabetes Educator* (the journal of the American Association of Diabetes Educators) found that orange juice and Coca-Cola affect blood glucose exactly the same. What that means is that you should eat the whole piece of fruit instead of drinking juices. (Yes, I mean "no sugar added" juices as well; Mother Nature has already added the sugar.)

The sum total of all this is that a little sugar is not necessarily a problem for the person with diabetes. You can have goodies such as low-sugar cookies (animal cookies, vanilla wafers, gingersnaps, etc.), low-sugar cakes with no icing (Cool Whip makes a great topping for cake or cupcakes), or low-sugar frozen yogurt or ice cream. Surprisingly, even a doughnut only has 25 grams carbohydrates, compared to a bagel's 75 grams. So a little sugar may be better than the no-sugar bagel. The doughnut has 10 grams of fat, so you wouldn't want to live on a diet of only doughnuts, but knowing you can have one once in a while means you don't have to eat a whole dozen at once.

Glycemic Index

June and Barbara: We might mention here, too, that the American Diabetes Association is definitely in accord. They say it's okay to have sugar if you limit yourself to no more than 10 percent of your total carbohydrate calories.

Getting back to the glycemic index, Table 4.1 shows that some complex carbohydrates are more complex than others and don't send blood sugar up as fast as mashed potatoes do. In this group are things like apples, sweet potatoes, black-eyed peas, and all kinds of beans. These are the "slow" carbohydrates, the ones that should help you keep your blood sugar more stable. Incidentally, Virginia, they're the very foods you've been telling us we should make the largest part of our meals—veggies and whole fruit.

The big problem we've always found with the glycemic index is that it only analyzes a small selection of carbohydrate foods and that leaves the majority of carbohydrates out there in mysteryland. That's why many dietitians say you have to test out individual carbohydrates on yourself and see which ones cause you to have normal or abnormal blood sugar. In other words, you create your own glycemic index by checking your blood sugar level after eating a portion of a particular carbohydrate food. That way, you can learn to predict the potential effect of foods on blood glucose and plan accordingly.

Virginia: That reminds me that the glycemic index rates pasta as a good carbohydrate. I've had some patients say they can eat a lot of pasta and not have a problem, but others say it really raises their blood glucose. I think I know the answer. The more you cook your pasta, the more you make it quickly digestible. Boiling too long changes the starch of pasta to sugar. So you need to cook it al dente in the true Italian manner and keep the portion small, such as one cup.

Table 4.1 • Glycemic Index

This index compares the extent to which different carbohydrate foods raise blood sugar. Since glucose raises it the highest and fastest, it is assigned the index number of 100. The lower the number, the less impact the food has on raising blood glucose levels.

Simple Sugars		Fruits	
Fructose	20	Apples	39
Sucrose	59	Oranges	40
Honey	87	Orange juice	46
Glucose	100	Bananas	62
		Raisins	64

Starchy Vegetables		Pasta, Corn, Rice, Bread	
Sweet potatoes	48	Whole wheat pasta	42
Yams	51	White pasta	50
Beets	64	Sweet corn	59
White potatoes	70	Brown rice	66
Instant potatoes	80	White bread	69
Carrots	92	Whole wheat bread	72
Parsnips	97	White rice	72

Dairy Products		Breakfast Cereals	
Skim milk	32	Oatmeal	49
Whole milk	34	All-Bran	51
Ice cream	36	Swiss muesli	66
Yogurt	36	Shredded wheat	67
		Cornflakes	80

Legumes		Miscellaneous	
Soybeans	15	Peanuts	13
Lentils	29	Sausages	28
Kidney beans	29	Fish sticks	38
Black-eyed peas	33	Tomato soup	38
Garbanzos	36	Sponge cake	46
Lima beans	36	Potato chips	51
Baked beans	40	Mars bars	68
Frozen peas	51		

June and Barbara: That's the way pasta tastes best, anyway. Now we need to know how long it takes different foods—protein and fat, as well as carbohydrate—to cause a rise in blood sugar.

Virginia: Carbohydrate foods will cause a blood glucose peak about an hour after a meal. Only a little of the calories from protein convert to glucose, and they're released into the bloodstream over a period of four to eight hours after a meal—at least that was the standard belief held by dietitians. But research done by Peters and Davidson reported in the *American Journal of Clinical Nutrition* (1993) shows that the glucose responses to meals with carbohydrate only, to meals with carbohydrate plus protein, and to meals with carbohydrate plus fat differ very little. In fact, only the fat-added meal showed a slight delay in glucose rise, but it was too small to be considered significant. Fats don't cause a blood glucose rise by themselves. In some type 2s, they don't tend to cause an increase in glucose, but in other type 2s, where the body doesn't use glucose very well, the cells tend to use fat as a fuel source more easily, and therefore the glucose from the meal tends to be increased in the bloodstream because it is not being used by muscle cells (our old friend insulin resistance is at work here).

What you need to do to get a reasonable rise in glucose after a meal is to eat a balanced meal—carbohydrate plus some protein plus some fat (less than 30 percent of calories in fat). Considering the above peaking schedule for different kinds of nutrients, we can get a good postmeal level if we add lots of fiber besides the protein and the fat. Don't get me wrong about protein. I'm not suggesting a high-protein diet.

You can plan on one to two ounces of protein at breakfast, one or two to three ounces at lunch, and three to four ounces at dinner. This is a fairly low-protein diet, but by including a little protein with each meal, lots of vegetables both raw and cooked, and starches with fiber (brown rice, baked potato with skin), you get a better after-meal glucose: type 2s get improved utilization of glucose by increasing insulin sensitivity, and you get satisfied so that you don't have to "eat the house down" later.

June and Barbara: We've heard that when you're trying to lose weight, it's not a good idea to drink your calories. Liquids slip down too easily, and since you don't get any chewing satisfaction from them, you may feel hungry and go off and eat a lot more calories in some more substantial form.

Virginia: Yes, it's my philosophy never to drink calories. You can have so many good things like all those diet soft drinks that are calorie-free, so why waste your calories on liquids? Also, liquid sugar absorbs so fast that you can't even cover it with insulin to get a decent blood sugar reading. We tell our patients to avoid *all* fruit juices and eat the fruit instead. Did you know that you have to smash eight apples to get just a half cup of juice, and then you've thrown away the best part—the fiber?

For people who are addicted to their juice in the morning, we suggest Crystal Lite's citrus blend flavor. It tastes like orange pineapple juice and it has no calories. My personal favorite flavor is the pink grapefruit.

June and Barbara: How do you feel about getting liquid calories via alcohol? We don't want to be accused of advocating drinking, but we feel it's our duty to acknowledge the big media blitz about the French paradox of two glasses of red wine a day lowering cardiovascular risk and increasing HDL ("good" cholesterol). Not long after that revelation, we read in *Diabetes Care* (April 1992) about a new study from Bordeaux, France, which showed that two glasses of wine with a meal have no adverse effect on glycemic control in people with diabetes. In fact, there was a slower rise in glucose after the meal in non-insulin-dependent type 2s than if they had water with their meal instead of wine. So you'd better hurry up and tell us what's wrong with drinking before the French lead us down the wrong path.

Virginia: A lite beer or glass of dry wine with a meal is no big deal, but if you do serious drinking, you'll probably find that it does serious damage to blood sugar control. You should never drink alcohol on an empty stomach because your liver gets preoccupied with the alcohol and forgets to put glucose back into the blood when your blood sugar starts getting low. That's why people on pills or insulin are always advised to have their drink with a snack or meal.

It's important to remember, though, that there are 7 calories per gram of alcohol, just 2 calories less than fat. A three-ounce glass of dry wine has 70 calories. If weight is a problem, you need to take that into consideration before you start following the French paradox prescription. And, of course, with hard liquor you should use only sugar-free mixes. Better still, use sugar-free mixes without the alcohol.

June and Barbara: We've often heard from dietitians that type 1s need to count carbohydrates and type 2s need to count calories. Is that true?

Virginia: True, but we teach both types to count carbs. For type 1s, we teach people who are learning to use Humalog or regular insulin to count carbohydrates so they'll know how much insulin they need to take to balance their blood sugar. As I said before, we use a formula of one unit of Humalog or regular insulin for each 10 to 15 grams of carbohydrate in order to get a good after-meal blood sugar. But it is important for each individual to test about an hour after a meal so that they can determine their own insulin-to-carbohydrate formula.

June and Barbara: What about the so-called dietetic and diabetic foods? Of late we've noticed that there are mail-order food companies that handle nothing but special sugar-free sweets and treats for people with diabetes. Are they good for you and worth the usually inflated prices?

Virginia: These candies, cookies, jams, and other items are usually made without sugar or their main enticement is that they're low in calories. I've heard dietitian Beverly Spears talk about these a number of times. She gives a lesson in label reading. Look at a label that says "no sugar added" and see how the product is sweetened; you may find concentrated fruit juice or something like corn syrup, neither of which is sugar but has the same effect on blood glucose. The number of calories will often be no different from regular food. We often see this in cookies, especially. Dietetic cookies may have 30 calories apiece, just like regular cookies and at twice the price. We recommend eating regular cookies that are low in fat and sugar, such as gingersnaps, vanilla wafers, animal cookies, or plain little shortbreads. Read the labels. Find a cookie that has less than 2 grams of fat per serving (which may be from two to six cookies, depending on the size). These are going to be much lower in price than dietetic varieties and cause little or no rise in blood sugar.

The other group of foods to watch out for are dietetic candies. Most times these are sweetened with sorbitol, mannitol, or other substances with "ol" on the end. They all have a laxative-like effect. Hard candies or chocolates with mannitol or sorbitol as their sweetener will have fewer calories than regular sugar candies, because they are a little lower in fat. It's not the sugar that makes the difference, because sorbitol and mannitol sweeteners have about the same number of calories as sugar. But for some people, a very little bit of this type of product causes severe gas cramps and possibly diarrhea. (The last thing you want to do on a long trip is give your child a pack of Velamints with sorbitol.) Sometimes caramel corn or other specialty products advertised for people with diabetes are also sorbitol sweetened. These dietetic products cost more, and we don't think they're worth it. We like to teach the person with diabetes to have some sweets containing a little bit of sugar. A tad of sugar is no problem in a well-balanced diet. Shop in regular markets and buy regular foods, not what's in the special sections of dietetic foods.

One of the interesting tidbits Beverly Spears discovered is that good old New York–style cheesecake does not cause much of a glycemic rise. That's because it's all fat and very little sugar. Some of us can't tolerate the calories of eating cheesecake very often, but for those who don't have a weight problem and especially for pregnant gals, this is a great alternative to eating cake. For Thanksgiving, they can have pumpkin cheesecake. For the baby shower or other special occasion, they can have a small piece of cheesecake and feel like they're having a really yummy dessert without raising their blood sugar much.

Fiber

June and Barbara: You've mentioned that fiber can slow down the rise in blood glucose after a meal. Dr. James Anderson, author of *Diabetes: A Practical New Guide to Healthy Living,* has long advocated a diet high in complex carbohydrate and fiber (HCF diet) for people with type 2 diabetes. His maintenance diet for overweight people with diabetes calls for 50 grams of fiber a day for a 2,000-calorie plan. The American Diabetes Association recommends that the diet include up to 40 grams of fiber a day. Since most people when diagnosed with diabetes are probably eating only 10 or 11 grams of fiber a day, they're missing the benefits fiber can give them. And it's not all that easy to increase the fiber in your diet.

Virginia: To give you an idea of how difficult it is to get 50 grams of fiber, a serving of Grape Nuts (1/2 cup) has 7 grams of fiber, a 1 cup serving of Cheerios has only 3 grams, in 22g of carbohydrate and a serving of Rice Krispies has no fiber with 48g carbohydrate. You have to eat lots of vegetables, fruits, and beans to get 50 grams of fiber in your diet.

June and Barbara: Table 4.2 shows some of the foods that are particularly high in fiber. By including some of these foods in your meals you can start building up to your 30, 40, or 50 grams a day.

Try as you may, though, sometimes it just isn't possible to get up to that 50-gram level, especially if you eat a lot of meals out. We agree with dietitians who maintain that the very best way to get your fiber, as well as all your vitamins and minerals, is from the food you eat. We used to take a fiber supplement, but in recent years, we've tried to get our fiber from foods. Two good fiber sources that we plug into every day are Bran-a-crisp, a high-fiber, low-carbohydrate crisp bread with 3.5 grams of fiber, and La Tortilla Factory low-fat tortillas, which are made with 100 percent whole wheat flour, are 99 percent fat free, and each contains a whopping 9 grams of fiber. Plus, they're delicious. If you have trouble finding these in your market or health food store, you can e-mail or call them and they'll put you on the right track: La Tortilla Factory, www.latortillafactory.com, 1-800-446-1516; Bran-a-crisp, www.branacrisp.com, 1-360-574-3552 or 1-877-679-3553.

Table 4.2 • High-Fiber Food Chart
(Listed in descending order of fiber content)

Beans and Peas	Serving Portion	Grams of Fiber
Black-eyed peas	½ cup	12.4
Kidney beans, canned	½ cup	7.9
Pinto beans	½ cup	5.3
Split peas	½ cup	5.1
White beans	½ cup	5.0
Breads and Crackers		
Pumpernickel	1 slice	3.8
Triscuits	6	3.3
Wonder high-fiber wheat or white	1 slice	2.9
Cornbread, whole-ground	1 piece (78 grams)	2.7
Graham crackers (21" square)	3	2.1
Cereals		
All-Bran with extra fiber (Kellogg's)	½ cup	14.0
Fiber One (General Mills)	½ cup	13.0
Raisin Bran (Post)	½ cup	6.0
40% Bran Flakes (Kellogg's)	½ cup	5.0

Fruits

Raspberries, fresh	1 cup	9.1
Blackberries, fresh	¾ cup	6.7
Pear, fresh	1	5.0
Strawberries, fresh	1¼ cups	4.1
Prunes, dried	3 medium	4.0
Apricots, raw, with skin	4	3.5
Nectarine with skin	1	3.3
Orange, fresh	1	2.9
Apple with skin	1 small	2.8
Plums, fresh	2 medium	2.4

Grains

Spaghetti, whole wheat, cooked	½ cup	2.7
Rice, brown, cooked	½ cup	2.4
Popcorn, air-popped	3 cups	2.0

Vegetables

Artichoke, cooked	½ cup	7.6
Squash, winter, cooked	½ cup	3.6
Pumpkin, canned	¾ cup	3.3
Asparagus, cooked	¾ cup	3.1
Green beans, cooked	½ cup	2.8
Zucchini, cooked	½ cup	2.7
Broccoli, cooked	½ cup	2.4
Carrots, raw	1 medium	2.3

Virginia: High fiber in the diet has lots of advantages. Not only does fiber improve carbohydrate metabolism, it lowers cholesterol and triglycerides. As if that weren't enough, fiber may also contribute to lower blood pressure, and it can enhance weight loss in fluffy people.

You should eat a wide range of foods to include both kinds of fiber: soluble, such as oats, legumes, and fruits; and insoluble, such as wheat products and bran. High-fiber foods are low in fat and are very filling. If you get filled up on these good foods, you're less hungry and won't be tempted by a stray candy bar. The person who decides to try the high-fiber route must build up to it gradually and also increase fluids in the diet dramatically. High-fiber diets have social consequences, as a diet high in fiber will cause gas.

Fiber supplements appear to provide benefit only if your diet is composed of at least 50 percent calories from carbohydrates.

June and Barbara: What about dietary supplements of other kinds for type 2 diabetes? Magazines and newspapers are always coming up with minerals and vitamins and even herbs that they claim will improve or even cure diabetes.

Virginia: People with type 2 diabetes should probably add a mineral supplement to their regimen—one that includes magnesium and chromium picolinate, as these have been found to increase insulin sensitivity in many people. Another supplement to add is vitamin E, which has recently been found to improve lipid levels and decrease the risk of heart attack. Also, ask your doctor about taking a small dose of aspirin daily to reduce the risk of heart disease. These are simple but really important areas to watch, because cardiovascular disease is the major cause of death for us type 2s.

Snacking

June and Barbara: Since we like people with diabetes to have as much flexibility as possible in their lives, how about skipping meals if circumstances such as plane delays in travel might make it hard to come up with the right food at the right time?

Virginia: Yes, you can skip meals as long as you're not on insulin. If you take one of the oral agents, you might start feeling a little low if you don't eat. Usually you won't, though, because your body makes extra insulin only in response to meals. If you don't have a meal to which it can respond, your body won't make the insulin.

While skipping a meal once in a while is possible, it's really not a great idea because you may get too hungry and overeat at the next meal. Our dietitians strongly advise our patients always to get up and have a nice high-fiber cereal breakfast even if they feel like sleeping in and skipping that meal. Then have lunch. If you get hungry midafternoon, have a snack, something like fat-free yogurt— fruit yogurt that is sweetened with NutraSweet tastes great and is under 100 calories. Low-fat cottage cheese makes a good snack, as do raw vegetables with low-fat ranch dressing. And, of course, fruit is the all-time great snack. They also strongly advise having another snack at bedtime. The reason for all these meals and snacks is that by spreading your calories throughout the day, you're less likely to store as many of them as you do when you eat them all at once.

Let's say your total daily calorie intake is 1,800 to 2,000 calories. If you divide them into more frequent, smaller amounts, you'll be much more likely to use them as energy sources. If, on the other hand, you don't eat all day and then consume 2,000 calories at one meal, obviously your body can't make use of all that and actually stores a higher percentage of the calories.

June and Barbara: We always recommend that you eat like a cat, not like a dog. The difference between the dining habits of these two favorite animal companions was brought home to us once when we were going to be out of town and wanted to leave some food for a neighborhood cat who always made it a habit to drop by for dinner—and sometimes breakfast and lunch. We got one of those cylindrical containers that you can fill up, and as the cat eats, the food drops down into the feeding bowl. The feeder had a stern warning that it was to be used only for cats, never for dogs; if you used it with a dog, death might result. We asked the pet shop clerk why death would result if a dog used it. Was it that he might get his head stuck in the container and suffocate? No. The problem with dogs is, they don't know when to stop. If you put a whole container of food out, the dog will dive in and, as the clerk said, "eat himself into oblivion." A cat, on the other hand, will just take a few mouthfuls of food now and then throughout the day—and sometimes throughout the night. Seldom if ever do cats eat large quantities at once, dog style. This is why, although there are such things as fat cats, you see them much more seldom than you do fat dogs. Dog owners often have to put their pets on diets because with the dog's typical one-big-meal-a-day program, they store up too much fat.

Virginia: Yes, fat storage can be a hazard for all creatures great and small. But for a type 2 it's a big-time hazard. That's because what we're talking about is building more fat, and more fat means more insulin resistance, and more insulin resistance just compounds our problems.

You may say, "Yes, but I'm not hungry until I eat. Then after the first few bites, I almost go crazy with hunger and it's a struggle not to overeat. I don't want to go through that more times a day than I already do."

I understand that terrible hunger feeling from experience. It's part of the disease. Food gives you a big insulin surge that makes you ravenous. From my experience, though, I also know that if you spread your food over the day and eat something every three or four hours, you'll find that you're far more able to control your eating and maintain your weight than if you eat all your day's calories at one gigantic meal.

Riding the Radical Rapids: The Low-Carbohydrate, High-Protein Diet

June and Barbara: Now we're going to present the minority opinion we mentioned earlier in this chapter.

The low-carbohydrate, high-protein diet is controversial, to say the least. In fact, many health professionals—especially dietitians—find it upsetting because it calls into question everything they've believed—and taught patients—over the years. When we began discussing this diet in the *Diabetic Reader*, one dietitian wrote to cancel her subscription. Her doctor had forbidden her to read it because it raised her blood pressure so much—not *following* the diet, just *reading about* it. An even more extreme case was a dietitian who called us at the SugarFree Center. Barbara answered the phone. The woman said, "May I ask you a question?" "Of course!" Barbara merrily responded. "Why is it that you're promoting blindness in people with diabetes?" Whaaaaat? This shows how strongly people initially felt about it. It has gone on to become a totally acceptable and nonfrightening alternative diet.

But before we get totally immersed in the low-carbohydrate diet, let's talk about a much less controversial subject: carbohydrate counting. Keeping track of the exact amount of carbohydrate you eat at each meal is now being taught by many dietitians as a better way to manage diabetes. Why is carbohydrate counting so important? Dietician Betty Brackenridge explains that some foods have a much greater effect on your blood sugar than others. And the big factor is carbohydrate. Ninety percent of the digestible carbohydrate you eat ends up as blood sugar. Carbohydrate comes in the form of starches, which you get from foods like potatoes, bread, pasta, and beans; and from sugars, which you get from foods like fruit, milk, candy, and table sugar. Protein, which comes from meat, fish, poultry, beans, dairy products, and fats (which you seem to get from just about everything these days, but especially from butter, margarine, salad dressing, and fried foods), yields small proportions of glucose. The glucose that comes from protein and fat tends to appear in the blood sugar gradually, up to several hours after the meal, if at all, while the sugars from carbo-hydrates show up relatively soon after eating. So the amount of in-sulin needed to control your blood sugar after eating is closely related to how much carbohydrate you eat. This is true whether you take injected insulin or whether you depend on your body's own supply. What this means is that most people (maybe you're one of them) can do an excellent job of managing food intake for better blood sugar control by simply counting the grams of carbohydrate contained in the food they eat.

In *The Carbohydrate Counting Cookbook,* authors Tami Ross, RD, CDE, and Patti Geil, RD, CDE, point out, "the importance of counting carbohydrate has been apparent for some time. In 1935 the famed diabetes physician Elliott P. Joslin said, 'In teaching patients their diet, I lay emphasis first on carbohydrate values, and teach to a few only the values of protein and fat.'"

Do you agree with the benefits of carbohydrate counting?

Virginia: Yes, I like the idea of helping people with diabetes under-stand the impact of carbohydrate counting, and to a certain extent I do it myself. I also like the system devised by my friend and dia-betes educator Sue Perry in Santa Fe, New Mexico. In this plan, the type 2 patient is given a "budget" of the number of carbohydrate servings for each meal. The patient then uses after-meal blood sugar testing to fine-tune the budget. You might discover what your budget should be by starting very low with the Fast Fast (discussed at the beginning of this chapter) and then gradually keep adding carbohydrate until you see your blood sugar control start to slip away. Using that carbohydrate level as the limit of your budget, you can go from there. But, as the authors of *The Carbohydrate Counting Cookbook* suggest, "keep in mind that your tolerance for carbohydrate may change over time, so your carbohydrate goal . . . [is] not set in stone. Factors such as exercise, medications, pregnancy, weight gain, and physical activity can alter your carbohydrate requirements." So, I might add, can stress.

June and Barbara: One of the nicest features of carbohydrate counting is that it's so easy. You only have to think of one dietary element. Food manufacturers are now required to include carbohydrates in the nutrition facts label. And, since you only have to count "effective carbohydrate"—the carbohydrate that affects your blood sugar—you can deduct the amount of fiber in a product from the carbohydrate.

Virginia: That's why I always tell my patients you don't have to count carbs in vegetables because of the fiber amount. I tell them: "You cannot raise your blood glucose with broccoli . . . you will explode first!"

June and Barbara: Deducting the amount of fiber from the carbohydrate also lets you slip in a little more carbohydrate, which is always welcome. Several books are available to help you count your carbohydrates. If you decide that this way of eating is a lifetime plan for you and you want to be more meticulous about it, a good accurate gram scale to find the number of grams in a specific food item would be of value. For example, if you look up an apple in a carbohydrate reference book, you'll find it has 13 percent carbohydrate. If you weigh it on a gram scale and multiply the weight by .13, voila, you have the number of grams you'll be eating. We use the percentage chart in *The Pocket Pancreas* by John Walsh, CDE, and Ruth Roberts, MA.

When people start playing the carbohydrate counting game and see the effect carbohydrate has on their blood sugars, they start thinking about a lower-carbohydrate diet, which, in turn, tends to lead them toward the low-carbohydrate diet. In fact, some people who read the first edition of this book achieved such excellent results with your Fast Fast that they wrote to us asking if there would be any problem with following the low-carbohydrate diet principle. We take it you don't go for this plan, because in your Fast Fast, you start adding back carbohydrate just as soon as blood sugars go down to normal.

Virginia: I'll tell you why we don't recommend that you follow this kind of an extremely low-carbohydrate diet permanently. It hearkens back to the old Atkins weight-loss diet or the so-called drinking man's diet of the 1960s. It was discovered that if someone consumes less than 60 grams of carbohydrate a day, they go into a state of ketosis. That means they're burning their own body fat to convert it to fuel. Of course, they lose weight. The problem is that they're eating gigantic hunks of meat, as much as they want, and that increases their health risks. It increases some of the same risks that diabetes alone does.

A low- or no-carbohydrate/high-protein diet is dangerous on a long-range basis because it is by default a high-fat diet. Protein and fat often hang out together. They're inseparable buddies. With a high-fat diet you can get very high blood cholesterol and very high low-density lipoprotein levels, and both of these contribute to cardiovascular disease. Yet another risk with protein is that it's hard on the kidneys. Actually, any diet that eliminates major food groups is not a good lifetime solution.

We do not recommend that you adopt a diet that is extremely low in carbohydrate and low in calories for more than a few days, just long enough to get your blood sugars down. Some people can do a Fast Fast to control blood sugars. They feel real good and have lots of energy. I, on the other hand, will get a high level of ketones and am liable to go out and attack a wheat field. Many people don't tolerate it any better than I do. And, ketones make your breath smell funny.

June and Barbara: Those are very logical reasons to be negative about the diet. But we're glad you didn't perpetuate the mythical fear many people hold that the ketones people with type 2 diabetes develop on a low-carbohydrate diet would lead to diabetic coma. Dr. Calvin Ezrin (author of *The Type 2 Diabetes Diet Book*) and Drs. Michael and Mary Dan Eades (authors of *Protein Power*) point out in their books that the risk of diabetic coma is only true for out-of-control type 1s in ketoacidosis. The "mild, beneficial" ketosis of the weight-loss phase of low-carbohydrate diets is a normal stage of fat breakdown.

This brings us to the basic theory behind the low-carbohydrate diet for weight loss. Exponents of the low-carbohydrate diet believe that excess carbohydrate rather than fat causes weight gain in some people because it stimulates the production and release of insulin, and insulin is a potent fat-building hormone. Indeed, the trend toward more support for this alternative diet is gradually building up. Dr. Julian Whitaker, long a passionate proponent of the high-carbohydrate diet in his book *Reversing Diabetes*, in his January 1998 *Health & Healing Newsletter* reversed his "dogma" with this statement: "While I maintain my stance on the deleterious effects of excessive fats, new research has convinced me that excessive carbohydrates pose similar risks."

A doctor on the Internet's LC-Diabetes list avowed that "most M.D.s aren't up to speed on low carbohydrate, but because it is a radically different theory from current dogma, some inertia is to be expected." He said that you can find doctors who believe in low-carbohydrate diets and more and more are realizing "the inadequacies of the old paradigms." And more surprising, Alex Haas, author of *Everyday Low Carb Cookery*, said he understood low carbohydrate was being taught to some extent at Harvard Medical School. He added: "Unfortunately, there will be many folks who acquire type 2 diabetes and heart problems that could have been prevented had the word gotten out sooner."

Incidentally, Dr. Ezrin in *The Type 2 Diabetes Diet Book* manages to combine the best of both worlds. His is a low-carbohydrate diet that also controls fat intake, and his maintenance diet has more carbohydrate than many other low-carb diets. Since he's been in diabetes all his professional life—he trained at the University of Toronto, home of the discovery of insulin—he recognizes the fact that all people with diabetes are not created equal. Different folks have different carbohydrate needs and capacities, and the challenge is to find what your carbohydrate "budget" is.

Virginia: I agree, a low-carbohydrate diet can be very beneficial for folks with diabetes . . . but not a zero-carbohydrate diet for extended periods of time. By the way, the premise that most folks propose for the way no-carb diets work is wrong. Protein foods cause an equal if not larger release of insulin. You have to have insulin to metabolize both carbs and protein. Most researchers have found that folks on low-carb diets actually eat fewer calories overall. I think it is because they feel more satisfied with higher protein, fat, and fiber (veggies) in their diet.

June and Barbara: We also want to confess that we have both been on a rather stringent low-carbohydrate diet for five years. June went on it because she was having trouble controlling her blood sugars when her insulin of choice, pork Ultralente, was taken off the market. At about the same time, Barbara, who had put on close to ten pounds after a two-week pasta, pizza, and polenta festival of eating in Italy, decided she had to do something. That something turned out to be the low-carbohydrate diet. We basically followed Dr. Richard Bernstein's edict of 30 grams of carbohydrate a day. He divides it into 6 grams for breakfast, 12 for lunch, and 12 for dinner. He advises fewer carbohydrates at breakfast because so many people with diabetes find it the hardest meal of the day to keep their blood sugar normal. Following this plan, we tried to eat about the same amount of protein—enough to make you feel comfortable but not full—at each meal. And, we must confess, we just let the fats fall where they may. So far the diet has accomplished what we both wanted it to: June got her control back and Barbara got rid of her weight. (However, it will return as inevitably as the swallows to Capistrano if she goes to New York and can't resist the wonderful breads or to Italy where she can't resist anything.) The best part is that it hasn't harmed our cholesterol and triglycerides. Dr. Bernstein maintains that if your blood lipids (those two things we just mentioned) are normal—as ours were—prior to going onto the diet, they will stay normal. If they are high, they usually go down.

We describe our adventures on this diet in a ten-thousand-word special supplement in the 1998 edition of *The Diabetic's Book: All Your Questions Answered.* And, we also tell who has no business going onto it.

Despite our success on this diet, we are by no means recommending it to everyone. The mainstream high-carbohydrate, low-fat diet is much easier to follow in the sense that it fits better into the standard American (and Italian!) way of eating. Let's face it, any diet that virtually eliminates breads, rice, potatoes, pasta, pizza, corn, chips, and cereals rather cuts into the dietary staples everyone else is wolfing down. The mainstream diet will also make you feel more comfortable in dealing with diabetes health-care professionals, since many condemn the low-carbohydrate diet as being unhealthy, and they generally won't support you in your desire to try it. So, you will need professional support. This is also not something you should try on your own, especially since, if you take insulin or certain pills, it may cause precipitous drops in your blood sugar and you may have some special condition (kidney damage or gout) that contraindicates this sort of diet.

However, this diet may be a life preserver and complication preventer for you if you've honestly, sincerely, and conscientiously tried to follow the mainstream high-carbohydrate, low-fat diet and have failed miserably at it—both your weight and your blood sugars have remained high. You may have even been accused of "cheating" (that dreadful word) by those health professionals who should know better. You may have reached the conclusion that diabetes is impossible, and you're never going to be able to lose weight and achieve normal blood sugar, so you might just as well give up and go eat a piece of pecan pie à la mode. This diet may give you another chance at success. That's why we call it "the diet of last resort."

We've received letters from people with diabetes who were furious. Unlike the dietitian who canceled her subscription to the *Diabetic Reader*, their anger was not because they considered the diet outrageous and unhealthy. No, they were furious because "This is the only thing that's ever worked for me. Why has no one told me about it before? It must be some kind of conspiracy!" Which is why we insisted on telling you about it, controversial though it may be. It gives you another option in this disease of many options. Sorting through them and discovering the ones that work for you gives you infinite possibilities for success.

Virginia: We are not as far apart as you might think. I, too, have learned that controlling carbohydrates is the answer to good control. I don't prefer to go as low as 30 grams a day, but I do feel that each of us has to find the balance in our diet that gives us good blood sugar control as well as feeling satisfied all day and not consumed with hunger by constantly thinking about what to eat next. Everyone should try to determine their own carbohydrate budget. Most people will find that eating vegetables (green beans, broccoli, squash, not corn or peas) fills you up and doesn't raise your blood sugar. I think that the recommended 50 percent carbohydrate was never meant to be filled with starch. There is a vast difference between a half cup of potatoes and a half cup of Brussels sprouts. In fact, if everyone ate lots of veggies, they would find their blood sugars are better and their cholesterol improved, and they would feel full from moderate calorie meals. The carbohydrate budget that I start most women on is 30 grams of carbohydrate at breakfast, 40 at lunch, and 50 at supper. Most men can tolerate 40-50-60. Amazingly enough, they can have good blood sugars and feel good, too. Here's to veggie power!

5

Emotional Aspects
of Diabetes

My Enemy/My Friend

WE REMEMBER WELL THE DAY OF WEDNESDAY, JULY 29, 1992, because that was the day we picked up Mary, our new Scottish Fold kitten. That day was made even more memorable by a report we heard on National Public Radio's *Morning Edition*. It was the story of Larry Trapp, the Lincoln, Nebraska, Ku Klux Klan Grand Dragon and head of Nebraska's American Nazi Party. Trapp lost both of his legs in 1988 because of diabetes complications.

From childhood, Trapp's life had been consumed by hatred of all those who were different from him; Jews and blacks were his favorite hate targets. So it was only natural that when Cantor Michael Weiser and his family moved into Lincoln, Larry began a harassment campaign, calling them at all hours to deliver anti-Semitic threats.

Understandably disturbed, the Weisers contacted friends and

the police for help whenever these harassments occurred. But after a while, Michael and his wife, Julie, started examining their own feelings. They realized that they were the victims of hatred, yes, but they had also become haters themselves. They hated Larry Trapp.

This realization caused Michael Weiser to come to the personal decision that he was going to change. He was going to practice the love, understanding, and forgiveness that he preached in his sermons at the temple. Cantor Weiser says that in Judaism, "the highest thing that a human being can do is to make an enemy into a friend." But he acknowledged that most of us never do that. He explains: "We have an enemy so we either avoid that enemy or we fight with that enemy."

He decided that the only solution to the enmity he felt toward Larry Trapp was to become friends with him. To make that happen, he launched his own harassment campaign against Trapp—a friendship harassment campaign. He began leaving messages on Trapp's answering machine that tried to point him in the direction of love rather than hate.

One day when Cantor Weiser was making one of his regular friendship harassment calls, Trapp picked up the phone and started shouting at him to stop calling. Weiser ignored the shouting and said simply and kindly, "I know you're disabled. Would you like a ride to the grocery store?"

Trapp was quiet for a while and then said, "No, but I thank you for asking."

A few nights later, Trapp called Cantor Weiser and told him that he needed to talk. The cantor and his wife immediately went to Trapp's house. He confessed to them how lonely he was, and the Weisers stayed and talked with him for more than four hours. Trapp later said he had never met anyone who showed such love and caring as they did. At the end of their evening together, Trapp symbolically removed the two swastika rings he was wearing and handed them to the Weisers, saying he didn't need them anymore.

A few months later, Trapp converted to Judaism. When his health worsened—he was dying of kidney failure caused by the diabetes—Julie Weiser quit her job to nurse him full-time. During the last months of his life, Trapp spent his time meeting with people who were willing to rethink their racism, showing them how his life had changed for the better with love and without hate.

This moving story illustrates the Judaic principle of making an enemy into a friend. This is a principle that we all can and should apply to our daily lives.

Think about your diabetes. It's only human nature to regard it as an enemy that threatens and torments you every moment of every day. But, instead of letting yourself be consumed by hatred, try to turn that enemy into a friend, a friend who teaches you valuable lessons that you might not be able to learn in any other way, a friend who constantly pressures you to make changes for the better in your life.

In her article "Forever Set in Your Ways at 30?" in the *Los Angeles Times*, health writer Shari Roan reported that studies show that by age thirty or thirty-five, your personality is pretty much set for the rest of your life. Major changes are difficult to achieve and unlikely. There is, however, an exception to this rule: "Catastrophic events, such as developing a serious illness or losing a loved one, can change people."

Ms. Roan cited the example of Mark, a rock band singer who lived a wild and dangerous life that included taking drugs. When a van in which Mark was riding crashed, he was left paralyzed from the waist down. Mark now considers this accident the best thing that ever happened to him. It spurred him to get off drugs, go to college and on to graduate school, and then to launch into a successful professional career. As he says, "I don't think I would be here today if this hadn't happened."

In a study of people who had experienced significant events in their lives, either positive or negative, psychologist Richard G. Tedeschi at the University of North Carolina found that negative events are the ones most likely to cause people to make changes. "Negative life events are so affecting that they call into question a lot of the usual ways of operating that people have adopted. Only because they're so traumatic do they pull people off their usual path."

Dr. Tedeschi goes on to say that people who have been transformed by negative events "often adopt a different philosophy of life . . . they begin to feel that life is good and useful; they become more expressive, more empathetic and tolerant."

The strangest revelation of this study is that profound positive events don't change people dramatically. This is because positive events don't challenge our basic ideas about living and what life is all about the way negative events do. In other words, unlikely though it may seem to you at the moment, diabetes can improve your life more than winning the lottery. It can, that is, if you neither avoid it nor fight it but turn it into a friend.

In the following section we'll ask Virginia to show you some of the emotional steps you can take to establish that friendship and make it a long-lasting one.

—*June and Barbara*

Denial

June and Barbara: We all know that people have different emotional reactions to a diagnosis of diabetes. Some have a healthy fear of what might happen to them, so they go to work on this diabetes thing. They get medical advice—and take it. They read, go to support groups, and take charge of their own health. They may become healthier than they were before they ever heard of diabetes. This group, unfortunately, is by far the minority.

What most people do at first—and this is a common strategy of self-protection when we feel overwhelmed—is to simply deny the diagnosis. We hear the word denial a lot in modern life. "He's in denial" means that in order to function at all, the person must push whatever has happened that he doesn't like so far back in his mind that he doesn't even recognize its existence. For those of you who aren't familiar with denial, maybe this parable will illustrate what it's like.

THE PARABLE OF DENIAL

Once there was a man named George who deeply resented the fact that there was such a thing as gravity and that his life was so affected by it. He detested gravity from the very moment he first became aware of it when he was five years old. He was holding his mother's favorite antique bud vase. It slipped from his fingers and fell and shattered on the floor. He never forgot how upset his mother was.

He loathed the fact that snow and rain and hail and apples and everything else dropped down, never up or sideways. He hated tripping and falling and banging his knees—all because of that #$@%A&* gravity. George began to spend most of his time brooding about gravity and how it loused up what would otherwise have been a perfectly lovely world.

As time passed, his resentment got worse. He despised gravity and the restrictions it imposed upon him more and more until he finally could stand it no longer. He decided he was just going to ignore its existence. "I'm not going to let this gravity thing ruin my life," he announced.

From that day forward, George pretended gravity wasn't there. If he held a piece of china or crystal in his hand, he let go of it and ignored the fact that it fell and broke. Before long his entire set of china and crystal was destroyed. He dropped his dachshund puppy so often that it would no longer come to him when he called. In fact, the puppy would hide when George came into the room. Then, one day he was at work looking out the window of his office, which was on the twelfth floor. It was such a nice day that he decided he'd go for a stroll. He opened the window, stepped out, dropped twelve stories, and broke every bone in his body. He's now in traction in the hospital waiting for his bones to knit, with an elaborate pulley system holding up his limbs against the force of gravity.

The moral of this parable: you can't change a situation with denial, and you'll only hurt yourself if you try.

Denial in reference to diabetes is a word we hear constantly from the lips of health professionals. So tell us, what is your secret of helping people overcome this formidable barrier to coping with and controlling diabetes?

Virginia: I've just finished reading four Tony Hillerman books. They're wonderful stories about the Navajo people, and this question of denial reminds me of the Navajo word "horzo." According to Hillerman, horzo is their term for being out of harmony. That's how I think most people feel when they experience the news that they have diabetes.

I rarely meet anyone who is totally surprised by the diagnosis. Usually they have had a suspicion, or else they have suspected they had something worse than diabetes. Nevertheless, when the diagnosis is confirmed there is almost always a period of grieving. The grief is often related to the losses that they anticipate diabetes will entail. Many times these are losses they have heard about or maybe seen in family members with diabetes: loss of freedom to eat what they want, loss of being able to schedule their time any way they feel like, loss of health or limbs or sight, even loss of life.

We approach each newly diagnosed person differently, depending on circumstances. For example, if the person is a pregnant lady, we cannot afford the time to work through the grief in a leisurely manner. We must get her blood glucose under control immediately. Because we're dealing with the health of her child, usually the patient can muster the spirit and energy to assist us with the task.

Many people, without the motivation of a pregnant woman, react with anger. They're angry at having diabetes and sometimes take it out on the health-care practitioner who gives them the news—the old shoot-the-messenger strategy. Others simply won't accept the diagnosis. I've seen people go from doctor to doctor to doctor trying to get one of them to give a different diagnosis.

My approach is to support such people with care and information. I tell them that I have diabetes and have had it for eighteen years. This usually helps them see that there is life after diagnosis. Then I try to give them information on how they will be able to live with diabetes day in and day out. I allow people to be unhappy about diabetes. Nobody has to like it, but we do have to go on living, and if you control your diabetes, you can live with it better and easier and healthier.

I encourage people to keep coming back for appointments at our diabetes center at least every two weeks until we see that they have a handle on the situation. We only work on survival skills for the first few months. People don't remember any of the complicated stuff if we try to teach it to them while they're still in a state of shock over the diagnosis. People look as if they're paying attention, and they may think they're on top of things, but if you ask them later what they remember about the first month or two after the diagnosis, often they can hardly remember a thing. This is true of many stressful events in people's lives. Can you remember the funeral of a close relative? Details of a divorce? We realize that the diabetes diagnosis is a traumatic event in their lives and try to give them only simple steps to follow.

How do I know this? When I was diagnosed with diabetes, I tried to approach it the way I do most things in my life—intellectually. "If I just find out everything about it, it won't affect me." Well, it affected me just like everyone else—with denial, grief, and depression. Because I know how they feel, I always try to encourage people to go easy on themselves for several months, to give themselves a chance to adjust to the diagnosis, and to learn that living with diabetes is not as bad as they thought it would be.

After they've mastered the survival skills of diabetes (how to test blood sugar, take medication, and follow a simple diet), then we can move into the advanced course. We know when they're ready for this because they start asking questions. We also realize that we may have to repeat some of the information about survival skills at this time, because they were in a diagnosis trance the first time we told them.

Then we start them on our "In Charge" course. This is an ongoing program where we give advanced lessons in living with diabetes: for example, how to eat out, how to adjust medications, how to prevent complications.

At the conclusion of this course, most people are ready for scheduled visits to their doctor every three months, plus checking in with diabetes educators from time to time for some fine-tuning. We find that many of our patients come in for a visit just to chat about how things are going and to find out if there is anything new in diabetes management technology that they need to know.

June and Barbara: What do you do when you meet people with hard-core denial for whom your standard procedures don't work?

Virginia: Yes, we do sometimes meet people who can look at any evidence and only see what they want to see. For people like this, calling in family members or close friends may help. But sometimes we just have to wait them out and let them know how the disease is affecting them and give them plenty of space so that they can come back for help and still save face.

There's one young man we see in our practice that took us six months to get in for diabetes education. He was diagnosed with type 2 diabetes although he's only thirty-six. He came to see one of our endocrinologists because his primary-care physician had sent him. He was a very busy business owner and was upset that these doctor visits took up so much time. His mother has diabetes, and he knew exactly what to do without instruction—or so he thought. When he failed to keep his appointment with the Diabetes Network, we called and arranged a new one. He called and canceled. We arranged new appointments again and again. Again and again he canceled.

We finally got him to come in by arranging the appointment with his wife, who realized the importance of good control. To make sure he got there, she came to the center with him. Although it took many broken appointments to get him into the center and out of denial and on track, he's finally getting into good control. His wife still comes with him to the appointments, and the two of them will be starting the "In Charge" class in two weeks.

Motivation

June and Barbara: Right up there with denial as a major emotional problem in diabetes is motivation: trying to make yourself do the things you know you should do for your diabetes and your-self. Usually denial is a one-time thing and once you get rid of it, it's gone forever. But that need to keep motivated is something you will always have to struggle with. Just how do you keep yourself mo-tivated day after day, year after year, your whole life long?

Virginia: That's a tough one! Almost every time I go to a diabetes conference for health professionals, there's a session on how to motivate your patients. The problem with diabetes is it's relentless. It's there day in and day out. It never goes away. It never lets up. If you get disgusted and decide that you'll just forget about it for a while, it will sneak up and whap you up the side of your head to remind you that it's still there.

Attitude

June and Barbara: Well, since it is always there, and you do need to do all those day-in-and-day-out (boring!) things to take care of your disease, what can you do to make yourself keep up with it?

Virginia: You need to get the right attitude about it. You probably think, "I'm sick and tired of fooling around with this diabetes thing every day. I'm sick and tired of never taking a break from it." And yet if I were to ask you, "Aren't you sick and tired of having to eat and drink every day? Do you pick up a piece of fruit or a glass of iced tea and say, 'I just hate it that I have to keep putting these things into my mouth and swallowing them every day for the rest of my life!'" No, you generally don't complain about that. You don't complain that you have to go to the bathroom several times a day forever or that you have to brush your teeth after each meal. There are a lot of things that we have to do all the time that we can't complain about. That's where that right attitude comes in. We have to decide that our diabetes routines are a basic part of life, like taking baths and sleeping and breathing, and do them without getting all worked up about it. That way, instead of being an odious chore, they become almost automatic, and we can turn our thoughts to more pleasant things.

June and Barbara: It also helps if, instead of grumbling and muttering about your odious chores and how deprived you feel and other disagreeable things, you focus on what's good about your life, the things that make you happy—in other words, develop more of an optimistic attitude.

Virginia: That's my philosophy. I've always felt that taking a positive approach, seeing the glass as half full rather than half empty, seeing the doughnut rather than the hole, has been very important to my success in life.

But even though I'm generally very positive and optimistic, I have to admit there's one area in which I'm not. I'm a pessimist about optimism. That is to say, I'm not very optimistic that people who are very pessimistic will ever turn optimistic. In my experience people who see the glass as half empty and who only see the hole in the doughnut hardly ever change.

June and Barbara: This reminds us of something we once read in an autobiographical novel by James Kirkwood, the author of *A Chorus Line*. The title of the novel, *There Must Be a Pony*, was from a story about twin boys. One was an incurable optimist; the other an incurable pessimist. Their father, who was trying to give each son a more balanced perspective on life, hit upon a scheme. On Christmas Eve he filled one room of the house with every toy and video game a boy could ever dream of having, and put a tag with the pessimist's name on the door. He filled another room from floor to ceiling with equine excrement and put the optimist's name on that door. The next morning he told the boys where to find their presents. An hour later he came back to see how each had reacted to his gift.

The pessimist was sitting on the floor in the midst of all his toys, sobbing and wailing and miserable because he couldn't decide which toy to play with first. The optimist was laughing and singing and whistling, merrily shoveling all the equine excrement.

"What's going on here?" asked the father. "Why are you so happy?"

"Gee, Dad," replied the son, "I figure that with all this equine excrement, there must be a pony here somewhere."

Optimists we don't really want to change. It's the pessimists we'd like to do a little attitude adjustment with. Why do you figure it's so hard to get them to change?

Virginia: Maybe it's because there's no motivation for them to change because they keep proving themselves right all the time, and that gives them a kind of perverse satisfaction. The militant pessimist will also tell you that he's never disappointed. He thinks of himself as a realist and regards those of us who are very positive and who see things optimistically as perfect fools.

But the thing about being optimistic and seeing things in life positively is that you often prove yourself right. When I look back on my life I see that almost everything has turned out positively. I am where I am because of how things evolved, and I am happy where I am. How can I—or anybody else—say I'm not in the right place?

Once when I was introducing myself to a class and telling them that I had type 2 diabetes, a patient in the front row looked up at me and said, "Well, how do you like it so far?" And you know how you tell the truth when you're not really thinking about it? I looked at him and said, "Well, actually it's been a tremendous professional advantage." It's true. To me diabetes has been a positive experience in many ways.

June and Barbara: To us, too! We wouldn't have had half the experiences we've enjoyed and met one-hundredth of the wonderful people we now know—including Virginia!—without diabetes. We know of many people for whom diabetes has had a positive impact—people who wouldn't have become doctors or nurses or dietitians or exercise therapists or psychologists if they hadn't had diabetes and been determined to learn more about their disease and to help others. We even know two young women who found the loves of their lives through diabetes. One was a diabetes teaching nurse who met her husband when he called on her hospital as a representative of a meter company. The other love story is a bit more complicated. The woman had diabetes and it inspired her brother to invent the Medicool, which keeps insulin cool when you travel, hike, drive in the car, and even keeps it warm if you're off in the snow. (Come to think of it, this is a double diabetes positive—a successful business and true love!) At any rate, the woman and her brother had a booth at a medical trade show to demonstrate the Medicool. Working in the booth next to theirs was the president of a company making another medical product. Between exhibit hours, they all got to talking and the upshot is that she became engaged to the booth neighbor, and now they're happily married.

We're so fascinated with how-diabetes-brought-me-happiness stories that we're collecting them. If you come up with such a positive tale, we hope you'll write to us and tell us about it. Please write to us at 5623 Matilija Avenue, Van Nuys, CA 91401; e-mail us at Prana2@earthlink.net; or fax us at 1-818-786-7359.

But it's not just people with diabetes who need to have a positive approach and a spirit of optimism. Their friends and family members need that attitude, too.

Virginia: A good example of this is Cathy Feste, who is a diabetes educator as well as a person with diabetes. She tells the story about what happened when she was a child and in the hospital just after being diagnosed. She asked her mother, "What does it mean that I have diabetes?"

Her mother said, "It means that our family will all learn to eat better and we will all be healthier." We should all be so lucky as to have family members who take that kind of approach. It really rubs off onto the person with diabetes. All diabetes educators are inspired by Cathy's positive approach to managing diabetes both for herself and for her patients.

But still it remains a challenge for diabetes educators to take a person who is very depressed or who sees diabetes as a tremendous burden and turn this attitude inside out into a positive one. And it's an even greater challenge for the person him- or herself. This is one reason we screen all our patients for depression. We use the Zung scale, but there are many "quick and easy" tests to help a person discover if they might have a problem with depression. People with diabetes are more likely to experience depression in their lifetime than people without diabetes.

It's funny how life gives us gifts that we can use positively or negatively. It makes me think of my friend Marci Draheim from Cedar Rapids, Iowa. Marci is a wonderful diabetes educator and an accomplished musician. She writes and arranges her own music and uses the power of music to help people experience their emotions in a positive way. She expresses her feelings about helping people with diabetes with a beautiful ballad she composed, titled

"I'll Be Here for You." She is a perfect example of a person using the gifts God gave her to help others.

June and Barbara: Is there any way to effect an attitude change in depressed and negative people and get them to start using their own natural gifts in a positive way?

Virginia: It's no secret that helping other people is a key to helping yourself. I encourage my patients to get involved in the American Diabetes Association or the Juvenile Diabetes Foundation as volunteers. When you're working with other people and trying to help them, it's much more difficult to focus on how miserable you are yourself. So get involved, if not with diabetes, then with some other organization that interests you. Focus on doing something positive for other people. I guarantee it will drive a lot of the negative out of your own life.

Finally, I have to say to discouraged people with diabetes: lighten up and don't be so serious about it. Maybe right now diabetes is on the front page of the newspaper of your life. It's not something that will ever get out of the news, but it can certainly be moved back to the lifestyle section or maybe even the comics page. It certainly doesn't need to be forever printed in bold front-page headlines like Bomb Explodes! or World Comes to an End!

Family and Friends

June and Barbara: It's often said that diabetes is a family disease in the sense that it has an impact on the entire family, not just the person who has it. Just what goes on in families when diabetes raises its ugly head?

Virginia: The way I put it is: people don't have diabetes, families have diabetes. Diabetes affects the entire family and may change the relationships and communication patterns among all family members. Family members may experience the same fears and anxieties as the person with diabetes—sometimes even more intensely. To add to that negative, the person with diabetes may feel as though he or she has a "low position" in the family and has no right to expect family support or assistance with diabetes-related routines or crises. Conversely, the person with diabetes may feel a role diminishment or power dilution if the rest of the family is handing out advice and instruction on his or her daily activities.

The situation grows even worse when the person with diabetes decides to protect the family from the stresses of diabetes by keeping the disease private and not allowing any family participation. Or the person with diabetes may not allow the other members any involvement by simply ignoring the hazards of out-of-control diabetes and doing nothing much to manage it. If the family and the person with diabetes have an unspoken pact to ignore diabetes management, they become "coconspirators" in the diabetes denial racket. The family members without diabetes may encourage the person with diabetes to go off the prescribed diet with tempting goodies or by planning activities that make it difficult or impossible to stay on the regimen. People with diabetes will participate in this racket, because it's then possible for them to temporarily allay nagging thoughts about their inability to participate in activities like other people. It's as if they think they can avoid feeling the pain and fear of complications and possible loss of life. But in fact, diabetes cannot be ignored. Denial of fears and failure to communicate feelings just cause more stress and emotional pain for everyone concerned.

I can't emphasize too strongly that enlisting your family

members in active participation with diabetes management is the first step to good control.

June and Barbara: That may not be easy to do. We've seen husbands and wives really irritated because one or the other has diabetes. Sometimes they resent diabetes and all the expense and trouble it can cause. One spouse can be extremely critical because the other cannot seem to handle diabetes well. Occasionally we've witnessed loud family arguments over aspects of diabetes, real knock-down, drag-outs in public. So how do you go about creating good, positive family involvement?

Virginia: There are several important steps:

1. Give your family permission to participate in your diabetes management. This is the step most often neglected and the primary reason people don't receive support. Sharing your life together means sharing the difficulties as well as the joys. Invite other family members to participate in diabetes activities, such as support groups, education classes, and diabetes association meetings. Remember that an invitation can be accepted or declined. Do not be judgmental about this.

2. Let your family members openly communicate their feelings. All members of the family must have the opportunity to express their fears and anxieties about diabetes, its complications, the restrictions of diabetes management, and especially their feelings about activities they may find upsetting or repugnant, such as blood glucose monitoring or shots. Just getting people to openly express their feelings helps diminish the impact of those feelings.

3. Everyone in the family needs to learn the principles of diabetes management in order to give effective support. The

whole family needs to get as much education about diabetes as possible. Each person needs a realistic understanding of what to expect from diabetes and what to do to ensure the best possible outcome.

4. You can make everything more comfortable for everyone, including yourself, by accepting diabetes rather than denying it. If you can't accept your diabetes, you'll find it difficult to accept support from others. Being in a position of disease with diabetes leads to a constant feeling of not being okay, so your self-concept is diminished. Acknowledge that you're an okay person, a good person, and that diabetes is not a reflection of who you are. If you have a feeling of being at fault about having diabetes, this guilt and anguish will color all your relationships and interactions with others.

5. Listen to love! You should actively translate the comments and suggestions about your diabetes management made to you by your family members as expressions of love and caring. That's what they are. If your family didn't care about you, they wouldn't bother to comment on your diabetes activities at all. You can transform your relationships by reinterpreting what may have appeared to you as annoying criticisms into what such comments truly are: expressions of love and concern. This is what any psychologist will tell you, and I know it to be true.

Stress

June and Barbara: It's impossible, as you know, to talk about feelings and emotions without talking about stress. And stress, as any experienced person with diabetes knows, can play havoc with blood sugar. June was once stunned when she found out that facing a particularly worrisome situation caused her blood sugar to shoot up from around 100 to over 200 in less than fifteen minutes.

Virginia: I could write an entire chapter on stress and diabetes, because it's such a knockout punch to blood sugar control.

June and Barbara: Why don't you start out by defining stress so we'll all be perfectly clear on what it is?

Virginia: Stress is any change in your environment that causes the body to activate its stress response and release stress hormones. These hormones are meant to rev up your energy so you can fight or run from the threat. This is the well-known fight-or-flight response to danger that is left over from primitive times when there were all those lions and tigers out there, not to mention lots of club-wielding two-footed enemies. What happens is the adrenal glands are alerted and they cause the release of glucagon (the opposite hormone from insulin; it raises blood sugar). Glucagon in turn signals the liver to release its stored glucose. This extra glucose is what causes the problem for us people with diabetes, because we can't make enough insulin to match the highly increased glucose levels. That's why June's blood sugar shot up like that. Her injected insulin wasn't enough to cover the extra glucose triggered by the unanticipated stressful event.

June and Barbara: What kinds of events and emotions cause this fight-or-flight response?

Virginia: Both physical stresses and emotional stresses activate the response. Illness, pain, infection, surgery, pregnancy—all these physical stresses raise blood glucose because of the release of stress hormones in the body. Probably more common in our daily lives, though, are the emotional stressors like work pressure, family problems, fights with your mate, money difficulties, hurricanes and earthquakes, and the endless upsets and crises people face in modern life.

June and Barbara: Some people seem to be under constant stress because they have a lawsuit pending, or are in the midst of a divorce or child custody fight, or are trying to care for an elderly parent and take care of their children at the same time, and so on. We have found, too, that diabetes itself causes plenty of stress in most people's lives. Wouldn't you agree that diabetes is another constant stress?

Virginia: I couldn't agree more. Ordinary events that aren't stressful for people without diabetes become major emergencies for the person with diabetes—things like, "Dinner will be late this evening," or "Your suitcase hasn't arrived with the rest of the plane's luggage." At any moment of the day you can find something that interferes with what you're supposed to be doing for your diabetes at that particular time. Tests showing high blood sugars can generate all kinds of fear: fear of blindness, kidney failure, or foot amputation. Not having the money to afford the test strips causes stress. I could go on and on. That's why at the Diabetes Network we teach our patients about the damaging effects of stress and how to change their response to it with stress management strategies.

June and Barbara: Ever since we wised up about stress and its effects on health, we've been working on ways to handle it. In fact, our *Diabetic's Total Health and Happiness Book* is full of stress-reducing techniques, from exercise, meditation, and visualization to such far-out methods as pets, travel, laughter, and hugs. Let's hear your antistress ideas, Virginia, as life in the twenty-first century looks as if it's going to feature new and weird stresses that we've never encountered before. We all need to be acquainted with every form of stress therapy that's been invented—and then some.

Virginia: I'm glad you realize you can't avoid stress, and therefore the more you practice the management strategies that work for you, the better. Here are my ideas on how to help yourself come to grips with stress:

Reduce the Frequency of Stressful Incidents

1. Make changes in family, social, and work commitments. Find activities that provide pride of accomplishment and satisfaction.
2. Set attainable goals and reasonable expectations so that disappointments do not become major stress points.
3. If you take insulin, learn to adjust your diabetes regimen and lifestyle so that the likelihood of severe insulin reactions is lessened; always carry glucose tablets and snacks.

Reduce the Intensity of the Stress Response

1. Learn conscious relaxation and practice it regularly (see the conscious relaxation exercise that follows).
2. Use meditation or prayer.
3. Decrease consumption of stimulants such as caffeine and nicotine.

Increase Physical Activity

Exercise reduces stress by relaxing muscle tension and increasing cardiovascular function.

Focus Your Energy

1. Identify the areas in your life that consistently result in frustration.
2. Control what can be controlled, and accept what can't be controlled. Remember, it's easier to ride a horse in the direction it's going.
3. Take action! Set your priorities. List tasks and break them into manageable sizes. Be realistic and flexible about time frames to achieve your goals.

CONSCIOUS RELAXATION EXERCISE

Practice this exercise in a comfortable place with little likelihood of interruption. If you fall asleep doing the exercise, as some people do, plan for awakening, if you're doing this on a short time frame (such as a lunch break at work). Get into a comfortable seated or lying position without crossing your arms or legs. Read over the exercise and then do it for yourself, using a similar scenario, or read it onto a tape and play the tape back. You may want to put your favorite relaxing music on the tape as well. Similar types of relaxation exercises are available on commercially recorded tapes.

Start this exercise by taking a deep breath . . . and letting it out very slowly. Feel the tension going out with the air. Throughout your busy day, deep breathing can be a quick and effective relaxation exercise. Put a small dot of colored tape on your clock at work and let it be a reminder to you that every time you look at the clock you will take two deep breaths.

Take another deep breath and as you let the air out slowly, allow your eyelids to gently close. Feel your body settle into your chair and get very comfortable where you're sitting or lying. Now you will begin relaxing by talking to the muscles of your body and allowing them to get completely relaxed. Start at your head. Feel the muscles of your scalp getting very relaxed. Your head will begin to feel warm and relaxed and your forehead will relax. Notice that your face is relaxing and smoothing out as you feel the tension leaving your muscles. Also take note of the relaxed warm feeling moving around to the back of your head and neck and that your head is feeling heavy and relaxed. Allow your head to sink deeper into your pillow or chair or to fall forward on your chest as your neck muscles lose all tension. Feel a warm flow of relaxation moving all around your neck, into your shoulders, and notice your shoulders drop as all effort leaves the muscles.

Now take another deep breath as you allow all tension to leave your head, neck, and shoulder area. Feel the wave of relaxation moving down your arms as all tension in the muscles of your upper arms, lower arms, and hands now flows out through your fingertips. Your arms are now completely relaxed and feel warm and heavy. Feel the warm, relaxed feeling moving across your chest and into your back. You can feel the tension leaving all the muscles of your back and abdomen as you sink deeper into your chair. Now allow that warm wave of relaxation to move through your lower back and buttocks and into your thighs. Feel a wave of relaxation moving into your legs as all tension leaves the muscles and flows through your knees, lower legs, and ankles. All tension and effort is now leaving your body through your toes, leaving the muscles completely relaxed and warm.

Now take another very deep breath. As the air flows out feel a final wave of warm relaxation wash over your body from head to toe, removing any tension left in any muscles. Now we will get into a deeper level of relaxation by counting down to the deepest level of relaxation. You will get more and more relaxed with each count as we count from ten down to one. You will hear the cue words "calm and relaxed" often. These will be your cues so that at any time, any place, you can return to this same level of relaxation by saying to yourself "calm and relaxed" and taking two deep breaths.

As we begin the count, imagine yourself on a beautiful, warm day with the sun shining in a blue sky. You are lying on a thick, fluffy cloud. You are completely supported, your body is totally comfortable and relaxed. Feel the gentle rocking of this beautiful white cloud as it gently floats you toward your most favorite spot on earth. Begin floating downward as we count ten . . . calm and relaxed . . . nine . . . you are floating gently toward your perfect place . . . eight . . . calm and relaxed, deeper and deeper . . . seven . . . feel the warmth and gentle rocking of your cloud . . . six . . . calm and relaxed . . . five . . . you are floating toward the place you most enjoy being, it can be a real place or a place you have only imagined . . . four . . . calm and relaxed . . . three . . . sinking deeper and deeper into relaxation . . . two . . . see your favorite spot . . . you are more relaxed than you have ever been . . . one . . . you are completely calm and relaxed . . . your cloud has brought you gently to your perfect place . . . look around . . . you can see in detail how beautiful this place is. Look at yourself in this picture . . . notice how relaxed and healthy you look in your perfect spot . . . take a deep breath and say to yourself . . . "calm and relaxed" and know that you can return to this feeling of calmness and relaxation at any time by taking two deep breaths and saying to yourself "calm and relaxed."

Look at yourself in this picture and see yourself as healthy and happy and solving any problems you may have. You are now in a state of complete calm, health, and happiness. As you watch yourself in the picture you can see yourself getting healthier, handling all your day-to-day concerns with ease and grace. You can see that this feeling of relaxation will stay with you throughout the day.

You will now leave your special place, but your feeling of well-being and relaxation will stay with you, and you will feel refreshed and full of energy. You will become more and more alert as we count from one to four and you will be fully awake, alert, and relaxed and feeling wonderful . . . one . . . two . . . three . . . four . . . welcome back.

Sex

June and Barbara: Sexual problems are as much a physiological issue as a psychological one. This might be a good place to discuss the issues sometimes associated with diabetes, since they can have such an emotional impact on all concerned. Breaking with tradition, let's put the gentlemen first. Does type 2 diabetes cause impotence?

Virginia: I hate to be the bearer of bad tidings, but yes, it can. Studies have reported that up to 50 percent of men with diabetes over the age of fifty have some degree of impotence. In fact, after many other symptoms of diabetes have been ignored, impotence is sometimes the symptom that finally drives men to the doctor where they're first diagnosed as having diabetes.

The primary physiological cause of this is neuropathy (nerve damage). The nerves that serve the penis and are responsible for erection become damaged by many, many years of high blood sugar. This causes an inability to achieve and maintain an erection. As with the other complications of diabetes, maintaining normal blood sugars can prevent this. Naturally, it's best to prevent impotence, since it is understandably very upsetting to a man. His libido is still intact, but he is unable to perform sexually. This can be extremely distressing not just for a man, but for the woman in his life, as well.

June and Barbara: What should a man do when affected by impotence?

Virginia: The first step is to have an evaluation by a urologist, because there can be other reasons besides diabetic neuropathy for impotence and erection difficulties. If, after all the tests are done, the urologist ascertains that diabetes is the culprit and the problem is physiological, not psychological, there are some very good ways to help resolve this problem.

Among the best are the vacuum erection devices. With these, a tube is placed over the penis and air is removed to create a vacuum. The vacuum simply pulls blood into the penis and causes an erection. These devices are not very expensive, don't require surgery, and have been helpful to many couples. The cost is often covered by medical insurance, including Medicare.

Another system that some people have found effective is to use injections of a drug such as papaverine or phentolamine, which causes blood to be pulled into the penis and results in an erection.

The problem may be resolved with surgical implants, either inflatable or semirigid. Although some men and their wives have found these to be very effective, there have been serious complaints reported about them. Sometimes additional surgery has been required to replace defective implants, to remove them entirely, or to repair the damage they have caused. A penile implant is something that you should investigate thoroughly and not enter into lightly. The best thing you can do is talk to several men who have had one and see how it worked for them and what problems they encountered.

June and Barbara: Of course, all these devices may now be obsolete because of Viagra, Levitra, and Cialis, the anti-impotency prescription drugs approved by the FDA. They are the source of a hundred hopes—and hundreds more tasteless jokes. Could you tell us how they work?

Virginia: I'll try to stick to the facts without the jokes. An erection is caused by increased blood flow into certain internal areas of the penis. Viagra enhances the smooth muscle relaxant effects of nitric oxide, a substance that is normally released in response to sexual stimulation. This smooth muscle relaxation allows blood to enter and pool in the penis, leading to an erection. Although Viagra can be taken thirty minutes to four hours before sexual activity, it is generally taken about one hour before, so you do need to plan ahead. On the other hand, Cialis can be taken and then whenever you get urge in the next thirty-six hours, it will be ready to work for you. Some people like that because it gives them more spontaneity.

June and Barbara: We've never known of a drug that didn't have side effects. What are those associated with these medications?

Virginia: So far the ones reported include headache, flushing, stomachache, a stuffy nose, diarrhea, and mild and temporary visual changes such as altered color and light perception and blurred vision. Most men would consider these side effects a fair trade-off for potency.

June and Barbara: Most men wouldn't consider death a fair trade-off and almost as soon as Viagra hit the market, there were some deaths reported that seemed to be connected to its use. Could you explain some of the risks associated with taking these meds and who would be advised not to take them?

Virginia: Men who are using medicines that contain nitrates, such as nitroglycerin, should not take these medications because the combination of the two drugs may cause a dangerous lowering of blood pressure. As a matter of fact, several medications are known to interact with Viagra, so tell your doctor about any medications—including nonprescription ones—that you're taking to make sure they're not on the interaction list.

June and Barbara: Are these drugs covered by most health insurance?

Virginia: Yes and no. Some insurance companies pay for a limited number of pills each month. I understand at this time most medicare plans do not cover ED drugs.

June and Barbara: Is there any final advice for men considering taking impotence medications?

Virginia: This is both the beginning and the final advice. You should first have a complete medical history and exam to determine the cause of your impotence and make sure it's something that the medications can help. Also, some men with certain medical conditions such as sickle-cell anemia, leukemia, multiple myeloma, or an abnormally shaped penis may not be able to take one of these. Unfortunately, one of the things that has been discovered in the last few years that this drug has been available is that men with diabetes are more likely to be on the list of folks for whom it doesn't work. As many as 50 percent will find impotency medication is not effective. For the other half, however, it is a great drug.

June and Barbara: Now it's the women's turn. Do they also have diabetes-induced sexual problems?

Virginia: Yes, although they're much less common, or at least they're less obvious and less frequently reported. It also may be that women's sexual problems are taken somewhat less seriously by the predominantly male medical researchers. On top of that, many male doctors may not be as careful about asking their women diabetes patients about sexual problems as they are about asking men. In a commentary in *Diabetes Spectrum* (vol. 4, no. 1) by L. A. Bernhard, Ph.D., RN, it was reported that in a survey of physician members of the Diabetes Association of Greater Cleveland, 85 percent of those who responded said they routinely asked men with diabetes about sexual difficulties, but only 33 percent routinely asked women.

Another article in that issue of *Diabetes Spectrum,* "The Differential Impact of Diabetes Type on Female Sexuality," described a study that made a surprising finding. Type 1 diabetes was found to have little effect on sexual responsiveness and sexual relationships in women. On the other hand, type 2 diabetes had "a consistently deleterious effect on both the women's sexual behavior and their sexual relationships." The type 2 women "viewed themselves as less sexually attractive, were less happy and satisfied with their sexual partner and sex life in general, were less interested in and more likely to avoid sexual activity with their spouse, and were less likely to lubricate adequately and to reach orgasm. . . . Their sexual activity was less varied and, understandably, they developed dyspareunia (discomfort during intercourse) more frequently."

June and Barbara: And to think that people always consider type 1 diabetes the more serious and restrictive and devastating condition. Were any reasons given for this bad news for type 2 women?

Virginia: The researchers had a number of theories. One was that type 2 women may experience more of the autonomic neuropathy that prevents adequate lubrication. (The autonomic nerves are the ones that control the heart and blood vessel muscles and the glands.) Another was that type 2 diabetes may have a more negative effect psychologically and socially because it generally occurs later in a woman's life than does type 1 and disrupts long-established relationships. The husband has often been the center of attention in a marriage, and when the focus changes to the wife's diabetes, a certain amount of marital conflict results. On top of that, a type 2 woman sometimes experiences mood disturbances, especially heightened anxiety and depression that may decrease her emotional availability to her spouse. Still another hypothesis is that because type 2 diabetes usually happens at middle age or later and is often accompanied by a weight problem, some of the sexual problems may have to do with a negative self-image, which in turn is caused more by the problem of being overweight than by diabetes itself.

But before any of you type 2 women let yourselves get all bent out of shape over this research and start overanalyzing yourselves and possibly creating sexual problems that weren't there before, remember that this study was of a total of only fifty-five women (thirty-two type 1s and twenty-three type 2s) and certain aspects of the findings were in conflict with findings in other equally reputable studies. But most important, remember that as Dr. Bernhard said in her commentary on the study, "each woman is first an individual with her own personal characteristics, and she may not be anything like the group (type 1 or type 2) to which she belongs."

June and Barbara: Clearly, if the woman sees that her problem is a psychological one related to diminished self-esteem, then some kind of psychological counseling would be in order. But what if it turns out to be more a physical problem caused by that autonomic neuropathy you mentioned?

Virginia: Fortunately, this kind of neuropathy is not as common as peripheral neuropathy—the kind that causes pain and eventual numbness in the feet and legs—but still it can be quite troublesome to the woman with diabetes, especially when it interferes with her sexual function or enjoyment. There are creams and jellies, such as the KY brand, that can aid the lubrication problem. As far as the autonomic neuropathy itself is concerned, the only treatment we can offer at the moment is the ever-popular, all-time favorite diabetes panacea: get your blood sugars in control! There are some medications on the horizon that may eventually help with all kinds of neuropathy. They are called aldose reductase inhibitors. It's nice to be able to look forward to these, but still nothing beats that well-controlled blood sugar when it comes to combating neuropathy.

June and Barbara: This may be a silly question, but can Viagra be of help to women's sexual problems?

Virginia: It's not a silly question. In fact, as soon as Viagra was approved for men, research began on the possible benefits for women. Have any benefits been discovered by now? It doesn't seem to make a difference for women, but never underestimate a drug company's interest in doubling the market. But it's only fair that women should have equal consideration. After all, what's sauce for the goose is sauce for the gander. But since this is beginning to verge on a tasteless joke, we'd better move along to the next topic.

Fear of Insulin Injection

June and Barbara: Of all the intense emotions that assail people with diabetes, especially type 2s, one of the greatest is fear of having to take insulin injections someday. Since insulin therapy is the last resort for treating type 2 diabetes and many type 2s never have to take insulin, people can have months or years or even a whole lifetime to live with the dread of "going on the needle," as it's often called. They build up a fear that is totally out of proportion to reality. We should know because June experienced that fear for a whole year while she was trying to make it on diet and pills.

Of course, certain individuals actually have a true pathological terror of needles, known as "needle phobia" among psychologists. What words of comfort do you have for all those people out there living in various states of dread at the thought of taking insulin injections?

Virginia: Many of us who have diabetes and have taken insulin can tell you that it is the least of the issues of having diabetes. As far as we can see, the biggest issue is not about having to take insulin but about not getting to eat brownies. This deserves far more attention and correction than all the emotion and upset surrounding insulin.

Still, I have seen patients who avoid going to the doctor, avoid participating in their own health care, and try to deny their diabetes altogether over the issue of taking a shot of insulin. Granted, taking shots is not everybody's favorite thing to do. If you have been avoiding the doctor out of fear that he or she might say you have to take insulin to get in better control, let me tell you this is one of the biggest non-deals in America today. The insulin syringes are 30- or 31-gauge needles. That's about the diameter of a hair. Ninety-nine percent of the time, with good technique, you literally can't feel them going in and out of your tummy. (The stomach is definitely the best place to give insulin.) So having to use insulin is not an excuse for not being in good control.

One thing we point out to people all the time is that giving an insulin shot, if it hurts at all, hurts a whole lot less than sticking your finger to check your blood sugar. You want to get out there and find the needles that hurt the least and check out the special devices for shooting in the needle. (The effect of these is to give you perfect injection technique.) Try out all the new technology and take advantage of the goodies you find to make insulin injection easier.

I have a lot of patients who say they wish they'd gone on insulin much earlier because they feel so much better after getting their sugars under control. This improvement in the way they feel overcomes the minor inconvenience of having to give injections twice a day and drives the fear of injecting right out the door.

Adjusting to Loss of Spontaneity

June and Barbara: When you talk to people who are discouraged about the things they've lost in life—or think they've lost because of diabetes—what seems to bother them the most?

Virginia: Although they may talk about it in different ways, it all boils down to just one loss, the only real loss: the loss of spontaneity. That's the ability to do what you want to when you want to do it on the spur of the moment without having to plan ahead and make special arrangements. It can be as simple as spontaneously deciding you'd like to go out to eat in a restaurant and order whatever you feel like at the moment. Or it can be a little more complex, like something I observed a few weeks ago.

I was doing a diabetes program for a hospital in Midland, Texas. We all had a great time, but since it went on all day it was quite strenuous, and I was looking forward to getting a little rest on the one-hour flight to Albuquerque. But the plane had some seats that faced each other, unlike the usual airplane seating where everyone is facing forward and you can catch a little nap if you feel like it. Just my luck, I got one of those seats and a couple plopped down across from me.

This lady was bound and determined that we were going to talk. I mean, she was the original Chatty Cathy. She delighted in telling me that up until thirty minutes ago they had no plans to go to Las Vegas. (The plane was going on to Las Vegas from Albuquerque.) They just got home from work and suddenly decided, "Hey, let's go to Las Vegas for a couple of days."

"So here I am!" she said. "I don't even have any clothes with me. I didn't even have time to put any makeup on." She'd brought her cosmetics with her and proceeded to put them on right there in the plane. They planned to buy some clothes when they got to Las Vegas. These people had the money, the freedom, and the spontaneity in their life to do that sort of thing. We should all be so lucky to be in the oil business (pronounced "awl bidness" in my part of the country) so we could do just that—if we didn't have diabetes, that is.

Your limitation as a person with diabetes is that you can't just hop in the car, run to the airport, jump on a plane, and go to Las Vegas. No, you'd have to plan your supplies and your injections and your meals. But then, how many of us can jump on planes on the spur of the moment, anyway? We have jobs, families, and responsibilities that keep us tied down to a routine. Diabetes can actually be a positive factor to get us organized and stay in touch with reality if we let it.

June and Barbara: Yes, it's true, diabetes can organize your life better than any of those books or courses on how to bring order out of your chaotic existence. But if spontaneity is the biggest thing in your life, you can be spontaneous if you plan for it. That sounds like a contradiction in terms, but it really isn't.

People are always telling you to be prepared for any emergency. We're especially conscious of this in California with our earthquakes, but other states have things like tornadoes and hurricanes and floods. You need to be prepared with a kit containing all your diabetes supplies and snacks so you can pick it up and run if disaster hits. We once heard David Marero, Ph.D., a psychologist from Indiana University, speak on being prepared. His theory was, why just be prepared for terrible happenings? The same preparation works for wonderful happenings as well.

Suppose someone says to you, "I want to take you on a horseback ride up into the hills, and we'll have a picnic supper and listen to music and watch the sunset." Do you say, "Oh, drat! I can't go. I don't have my insulin (or pills or whatever)"? No, you say, "Terrific. I'll just grab my Spontaneous Happy Event Kit, and we're off."

We know a young guy with diabetes who practices what you might call modified spontaneity. He and a buddy pack their bags and his diabetes supplies and they go to the airport and take the next plane that's going somewhere no more than an hour or two away. His diabetes never causes him any problems—at least no more than it would at home.

So you see, spontaneity is possible. But, really, we've found that in the modern world, spontaneity is becoming an overrated commodity. Before June's diabetes diagnosis, we used to travel in Europe by buying a Eurail Pass and jumping on a train—any train—and getting off wherever the mood struck us. Then we'd wander around until we found a hotel room. No more. And that's not just because of diabetes. More and more people are traveling, and the hotel you decided to stay in is likely to be *complet* as the French say or fully booked as the British put it. Ditto for the restaurant you'd like to eat in. If you want to have a really great trip, you need to plan it as carefully as a space launch. That's what we do now, and guess what? It's a lot more fun than winging it. You get weeks and weeks of anticipation as you prowl through guidebooks picking out where you want to visit, corresponding with picturesque hotels in convenient locations, even reserving special restaurants ahead of time. By the time you get there you feel you know the place, and that knowledge sets you free to relax and enjoy yourself.

So if you prefer spontaneity or anticipation or a combination of the two, you can have it in most areas of your life. Diabetes won't stop you. We don't need to envy the "awl bidness" pair—except maybe for their money.

6

Paying the
Bill for Diabetes

Dollars and Nonsense

DEALING WITH THE FINANCIAL ASPECTS OF AMERICAN MED-
ical care these days is like walking into a madhouse, and it's beginning to seem like the most violent shock treatments are reserved for
people with diabetes. Your first problem is getting health insurance at all, because insurance companies are only willing to insure
perfect specimens. It's like the automobile insurance companies
wanting to insure only people who've never had an accident and are
statistically unlikely to have one.

It's not so bad if you live in a state that has pooled-risk insurance coverage available. Over half the states now offer this kind of
program. Pooled risk means that any insurance company that
wants to do business in a state must contribute to a fund that will
issue health insurance to those who would otherwise not be able
to obtain it or would only be able to get it for exorbitant rates.

225

They cannot charge more for pooled-risk insurance than 125 to 150 percent of the average health insurance premium in that state. Do you know of any other good developments in this?

If you have been rejected for health insurance coverage—either group or individual—you may be eligible for pooled risk, although check on the cost; it varies widely by state. Call your state's insurance commissioner or health department to find out the details for your state.

That's when the craziness begins. An article in the *Los Angeles Times*, "Working Without a Net," described what happened to a self-employed man with the preexisting condition of diabetes. When he quit his previous job to start his own business, the cost of private health insurance for himself and his wife started doubling every three months. When it hit $16,000 a year—just about equal to the amount of his annual income—he had to shut down his business and go to work for a government agency just to get the medical insurance to cover his diabetes.

The article also told of growing numbers of people who are hanging on to jobs they've outgrown or detest simply to keep their health insurance. It's not only bad for business to have all these unhappy (and therefore less efficient) employees, but it takes all the joy and enthusiasm out of the work life of the employee who is being held a hostage to health insurance.

Even if you like your work and have insurance, your situation still isn't totally sensible and sane. Each year you find your coverage eroding and your deductible and co-payment increasing. This is because medical charges are getting out of hand and out of sight. (The *Times* article gave the example of a woman who had a miscarriage and ended up with a $6,000 bill for one night's stay in the hospital. The bill included such charges as $14 for four ounces of mouthwash and $17 for a 15-cent sanitary pad.)

And the underlying reason for such exorbitant charges is the essence of nuttiness. Only around one-quarter of hospital patients have private health insurance. Therefore these people pay not only for their own care but for a portion of the care of those who have no coverage and those who have Medicare or Medicaid, whose payments, set by the government, are not adequate by hospital standards. This makes about as much sense as if you went to a restaurant for dinner and when you got your check, you discovered you were being charged to cover meals for three other diners who didn't have enough money to pay the bill.

The one bright light on the insurance horizon is a significant improvement in Medicare coverage for people with diabetes. In 1997, Congress enacted legislation to cover diabetes education and to provide meters and blood sugar test strips for all people with diabetes, not just for those who take insulin, as before. In October 1998, Medicare's revision for diabetes testing supplies stipulated that each person with diabetes's physician must supply a Physician's Order Form every six months in order for the patient to qualify for Medicare-covered diabetes testing supplies. Type 2s are eligible for one hundred strips and lancets every three months; type 1s receive one hundred strips and lancets per month. If you need more than the allotted number to stay in control, your Physician's Order Form must specify why you need to exceed the guidelines. Reasons are "documented episodes" of widely fluctuating blood sugars, recurring insulin reactions, and ketoacidosis.

This is a true breakthrough for type 2 people. Now we have Medicare Part D. This is the drug benefit portion for Medicare participants, so people with diabetes have coverage for supplies and at least some drug coverage as well.

We could go on and on spelling out the problems—and lack of

solutions—with health care. But better that we do as Barbara used to do when we were directors of the SugarFree Centers. If we were going out of town, she always left a list of phone numbers where we could be reached, so that others could "get in touch with us with the solutions to any problems that may have developed in our absence." So we'll ask Virginia to get in touch with you with solutions to the problems associated with the financial aspects of diabetes.

—*June and Barbara*

Health Insurance

June and Barbara: It would help if you could start with an overview of the kind of health insurance plans that are available, so we can understand what each has to offer.

Virginia: It's important for everyone to understand the different types of insurance, but it's vital for people with diabetes.

Many people have an insurance plan that gives them the option of choosing an HMO (health maintenance organization). For people who have a chronic disease like diabetes, these plans have advantages and disadvantages. One advantage is that if you require lots of medications, these programs usually allow you to get them for a nominal co-payment (the amount you have to pay out of pocket) of $5 to $10 for each prescription. A disadvantage is that they often operate under a formulary. This means that they have a committee that selects medications for their plan. They make their selections based on effectiveness and price. To achieve cost savings they will select one or two specific drugs from each classification instead of allowing physicians on their plan to prescribe a variety of brand names.

For people with diabetes, this means that you may not get your usual brand of insulin. This is one area in which I see many patients make a mistake. There's probably no difference between brands, and you should get whatever costs less. I've seen patients pay an extra filling fee just to get the particular brand of insulin they've been using. This can turn out to cost more than if they'd just forgotten about their HMO pharmacy service and gone out and bought the insulin retail. If your insurance plan says you have to pay a larger co-pay for a type of insulin not on the formulary, you should protest. If the brand they have selected as the formulary brand doesn't have the type of insulin you need, such as a long-acting insulin like Lantus, then the plan should make the other brand of the same type available at the formulary cost. Fight for it.

Another way people with diabetes can cause themselves problems is when it comes to buying syringes. Let's say you prefer a certain brand of syringe, yet the HMO will only give you a lesser quality syringe for your co-payment, and you think you're stuck with that. In fact, syringes are so inexpensive (especially if you shop around and find specials on them, and double especially if you reuse them four or five times) that you can buy them outside your co-payment plan.

Where your co-payment arrangement comes in handy is for expensive medications like those for high blood pressure. Those can be purchased with great savings on your prescription card.

Generic Drugs

June and Barbara: Sometimes this works well when you aren't even on an HMO. Barbara's mother, who has Blue Shield, can get her "maintenance" prescriptions for only $10 each if she buys them through a certain drugstore's mail-order plan. Of course, they prefer to give generics in this case, but if her physician insists, they will provide the exact drug prescribed.

We should mention some of the differences between generic and trade-name drugs. One of the best explanations we've seen is from Mike Voelker, Pharm.D., erstwhile pharmacist at N.M.C. Homecare in Southern California:

> Generic drugs [drugs not protected by trademark] are in demand today and for many valid reasons. First, insurance companies and other health-cost payment systems are encouraging their members to use generic drugs by offering people a lower co-payment if they do. Second, the FDA [Food and Drug Administration] is shortening the time period for trade-name drugs to become generic. And, third, over the next three to four years the federal government is phasing in Medicare payments for prescription drugs, and, just as many states do with their Medicaid programs, the federal government will probably demand that generic medications be provided whenever possible.
>
> For the above reasons it is safe to say that generics are here to stay. But, buyer beware! Some warnings are in order. Brand-name drugs and their generic forms are not necessarily identical. Switching to a generic without proper precautions may cause serious problems. To understand the possible difficulties, you have to understand what generic drugs are and how they're made.
>
> A generic drug has exactly the same amount of the active ingredient as the trade-name product. The active ingredient by weight, however, makes up only a fraction of the total weight of the tablet or capsule. For example, a Lanoxin 0.25-mg tablet weighs about 2.5 mg, but the active

ingredient, digoxin, makes up only about 10 percent of the total weight of the tablet. The other 90 percent comprises what pharmacists call 'excipients'—fillers, binding agents, coloring, etc. It is these extra ingredients that very often determine how much of the active drug is absorbed into the bloodstream and how quickly. In some cases, more drug is absorbed with the generic form, and in other cases less is absorbed. This difference can be very critical, depending on the type of drug.

With the following classes of drugs, you, your doctor, and your pharmacist must be extremely careful when changing to the generic form:

- Cardiovascular drugs (Lanoxin, Altace, etc.)
- Hormone and related drugs (Premarin, Synthroid, etc.)
- Psychotherapeutic drugs (Thorazine, Elavil, etc.)
- Anticonvulsants (Dilantin, Depakene, etc.)
- Oral diabetes medications (Glucophage)

A person with diabetes, for example, can switch from the trade name Glucophage to the generic metformin, but you should always ask your physician first. When the switch is made, you must be very diligent about testing for hyper- or hypoglycemia so that you can determine whether the generic is being absorbed in the same way as the trade-name pill. Then, once you have successfully switched, you have to make sure that you are always provided with that particular brand of generic because the same generics manufactured by different companies also differ in their excipients. This is another complication which means that only those in the know can protect themselves from drug overdose or underdose.

With classes of drugs not on the above list, such as antibiotics and analgesics, it is perfectly okay to switch to a generic brand without any special monitoring.

The final word on generics, then, is to enjoy the savings they offer, but make sure that you and your physician and your pharmacist work as a team to ensure their safe and efficacious use.

Voelker also told us that pharmacies actually make a greater percentage of profit on generics than on brand names, so if a pharmacist discourages you from purchasing a certain generic, he is doing so for medical reasons and not out of some sordid profit motive. By the way, there's another piece of good news about generics: sometimes when generics come on the market, the brand-name drug companies lower their price, so you can get your brand-name drug at a lower price.

But let's get off drugs and back to HMOs. What else do we need to know about them?

HMOs

Virginia: Another significant feature is that they use a "gatekeeper" system.

June and Barbara: What does that mean? Do they have someone guarding the door who won't let you in unless you can prove you're really sick?

Virginia: It sounds that way, but it's actually a system that requires you to select a primary-care physician (a family doctor or internist). This physician will have to write you a referral before you can go to see a specialist.

June and Barbara: Does this mean that you can't just march in and say, "I have diabetes and I want to see an endocrinologist"?

Virginia: That's right. And you can't go directly to an orthopedist when you have a back problem, or to a psychiatrist if you're feeling depressed, and so forth. The reason the HMOs do this is so that the specialists won't be used indiscriminately when a primary-care physician could have done as good a job. This makes sense. After all, patients aren't always adept at diagnosing their conditions and knowing what kind of specialist—if any—they need. It's also a cost-effective way of providing health care; but if you have a chronic disease like diabetes, it can become a hassle.

June and Barbara: It certainly can. We've talked to lots of people with diabetes who belong to HMOs. They know from experience when they need to see an endocrinologist for a diabetes problem, and yet they're slowed down by having to first see the primary-care physician and then wait for him or her to decide that the problem truly is something that requires an endocrinologist's attention, and then wait to get the appointment with the endocrinologist. All the while, the diabetes problem goes untreated. Is there nothing that a person with diabetes can do to keep this situation from occurring over and over again?

Virginia: Many HMOs in our area allow an endocrinologist to become a primary-care physician for individuals who have an endocrine disease. You should investigate and see if you can work out that kind of arrangement, because it gives you the best of both worlds: the care you need from your endocrinologist or diabetes specialist without the hassles of having to get a referral every time you need to see him or her.

One more thing you need to investigate when choosing an

HMO: look into what they cover. Do they cover your blood glucose meter and strips? The strips are probably the most expensive part of diabetes management.

Hopefully, you live in one of the forty-eight states that have passed legislation mandating that insurance pay for diabetes education and supplies. Our state passed this legislation several years ago, and it really makes a big difference. Insurance companies now pay for education (some more than others), and we have no more hassles over strips and meters. The only thing that is still a problem is the employee who thinks he has regular health insurance, only to discover that his plan is a "self-insured plan" by his employer. This special exception for companies allows them to fund their own insurance plan without regulation from individual states, which means they are not subject to the new legislation. We all know that the companies would be better off to pay for education and supplies and would save money in the long run, but they generally don't know that.

June and Barbara: That certainly is something to look into. We know of one young woman who was furious because her HMO wouldn't cover her meter and strips. Yet they would cover them for older people on Medicare because these people had signed their Medicare benefits over to the HMO and Medicare did cover meters and strips for them. The young woman resented the fact that she, who had a whole lifetime of diabetes ahead of her, was not provided with what was necessary to keep her disease in control, while the older people who had less risk of developing complications were. Obviously, it was more a matter of economics than concern for the well-being of the patient.

Another thing we have noticed about HMOs is that what is covered is often based on what kind of policy you have. Some people say, "I belong to SpendthriftCare HMO, so I'll automatically get everything covered." Others lament, "I belong to SkinflintCare and they never cover anything." In many HMOs, some members may have a policy that covers no meters, strips, or prescriptions at all. Others have to pay a portion of the cost. And some lucky devils in the same HMO get virtually everything free of charge. The kind of policy you have, of course, is based on what your employer (or you as an individual subscriber) pays.

When it comes to specific types of insulin, you may want to really get serious with your HMO and demand that they provide it even if the insulin brand on the formulary doesn't include it, such as the insulin lispro (Humalog). Be especially diligent when it comes to requesting insulin pens. Everyone in Europe gets pen-type delivery devices for insulin and they are more accurate and convenient.

Private Insurance

Virginia: You could choose a standard indemnity-type insurance plan. This is traditional private insurance. This insurance covers a portion—usually 80 percent—of the costs of hospitalizations and outpatient services, such as physicians and prescriptions, after you meet a certain deductible. The downside of this kind of policy is that most of the time you must pay cash up front and then get reimbursed, so it can lead to a lot of paperwork.

June and Barbara: We once read of a survey that revealed that the thing elderly patients fear most about going to the hospital is not death, but the paperwork they're going to have to handle. We may be cynics, but we suspect that most insurance companies make filing for claims so difficult and keep bouncing back your claims for little niggling details so that you'll become so frustrated and discouraged that you'll just give up and they won't have to pay. Ernest

Hemingway once said that if you want to be a writer, you have to be the world's most persistent son of a bitch. The same thing holds true if you want to collect on your insurance.

Virginia: There is an upside, though. With this kind of insurance, you have complete choice about the care you get and the physicians and hospitals who give it to you.

June and Barbara: But even this kind of policy, which we both have, is starting to "suggest" that you go to certain hospitals and physicians. They have contracted with these providers for a lower rate and the result is "a lower out-of-pocket expense to you." We always try to follow their suggestion, but even so, the out-of-pocket expense doesn't seem all that low.

Virginia: That's because of cost shifting, which you touched on in the introduction to this chapter. Since it's referred to so frequently by health professionals and legislators when they talk about the crisis in health care in this country, let me explain in a little more detail what cost shifting is and, more important, why it exists.

Your doctor or pharmacy or other specialist is receiving reimbursement from a variety of sources such as Medicaid, Medicare, HMOs, PPOs (preferred provider organizations), indemnity insurance, and that small category of people who just pay cash. When the doctor receives payment from Medicaid or Medicare, it's been discounted greatly. If his fee for an office visit is $60, he may be getting only $20 from Medicaid for that same visit. The local HMO may be paying him only $35. If you have indemnity insurance, you pay the full $60. Of course, you receive $48 back (80 percent of the $60), but only after you've met your deductible. The patient in the waiting room of an HMO will pay maybe $8 or $10 in co-payment for the visit.

In the past, indemnity insurance was the preferred way to go. But more and more patients with indemnity plans are discovering that physicians and health-care organizations have to increase their fees to them to compensate for the discounting that's taking place on the other plans—thus you have the term "cost shifting."

This cost shifting is getting to the point that the indemnity insured patient is having to pay a higher and higher percentage of the total cost of health care. Those of us who have indemnity plans or pay cash are subsidizing Medicaid and Medicare by more than just our tax dollars. We're subsidizing it every time we go to the doctor or hospital.

Am I saying this cost shifting and subsidizing is good or bad? Neither. I'm just saying that this is how it is. Do I think we need a national health-care system? I think we are getting closer to needing some kind of system that assures everyone of quality health care. I don't think the government has to be the one to deliver this care.

June and Barbara: But don't you think we need some kind of improvement in our health-care system? More and more people—often those with chronic conditions like diabetes—are falling through the cracks and getting no care at all, or else are going bankrupt from paying exorbitant medical costs, losing their homes, and then finally getting public assistance so they can have at least some kind of medical care.

Virginia: I agree that we need something, but first we have to do a much better job with our public health care. It would take so little money, just the cost of one or two heart transplants in every state, to pay for the immunizations that could save a zillion lives. If the money from three or four amputations a year were put into the cost of shoes for people with at-risk feet, it could save the rest of the amputations.

America's health-care priorities need to change. We need to put more money, effort, and concern into preventing disease, into taking care of the basics extremely well—basics like prenatal care, immunizations, and the prevention of chronic diseases.

No, I don't want to see a national health-care system like the much-praised one in Canada, where a person must wait two or three years to get gallbladder surgery because it's considered "elective."

June and Barbara: It's true that the other systems aren't perfect, and we would want America to do a better job. But can we? Good medical care takes money—more and more every day—and there is less and less of that commodity available in this country.

Virginia: Let me give you an example of how it can be done. At our diabetes center we have a pregnancy program where we work with women who have gestational diabetes and who have diabetic pregnancies. We have a team approach, where we involve the perinatologist (a doctor who specializes in high-risk pregnancies), the endocrinologist, and the nurses and dietitians from the Diabetes Center. We are able to manage these patients very effectively and monitor them closely and thereby prevent many problems of the diabetic pregnancy. We have normal-weight babies, healthy babies, babies who do not spend time in the neonatal intensive care unit. Yet with all that we are extremely cost-effective. And that's not even considering the long-range cost difference between delivering a healthy baby and an unhealthy one.

June and Barbara: But can this be done in a public health-care situation?

Virginia: Right now we're working with the Medicaid department in our state, trying to partner with them to help them do a better job of managing their patients in a cost-effective way. How is it working out?

That American Diabetes Association Recognition of Diabetes Education Centers Program provides a way for third-party payers to know where quality care is being given and to utilize resources more effectively so we get better care at a lower cost. Find a recognized program at Diabetes.org.

I think you may see in the future that the third-party payer, whether private insurance or public, will select for you the places where you will go for a certain surgery, your diabetes education, and other specialty kinds of care.

Pooled-Risk and COBRA Insurance

June and Barbara: If you have health insurance, but you don't feel that it gives you the kind of coverage you want, is there any alternative or, because you have diabetes, are you pretty much stuck with what you have?

Virginia: First off, you should remember that it's unlikely that you'll ever be totally delighted with your insurance coverage. No one has been since back in the time when some unions were able to negotiate contracts that included 100 percent coverage with no deductible. Those days are gone forever!

I must caution you to investigate very carefully and make certain you can get something else before you give up any insurance coverage. As previously mentioned, many people—especially people with diabetes—will find that they must select or hold on to a job simply for the insurance coverage that it offers.

Even if you're offered a different job that has good insurance and you would prefer to take the new job, you may wind up hanging on to the job you already have because the health insurance with the new company won't cover a preexisting condition for the first six months or a year or, in some dismal cases, as long as two years. If you have diabetes, this means your new insurance will be of little value to you during the preexisting condition exclusion period. After all, any health problem that you are likely to have may well be related to diabetes—or the insurance companies will claim that it is.

In 1997, the Kennedy-Kassebaum Bill was passed and was supposed to help people with the portability of their insurance. If you change insurance plans within a thirty-day period, you cannot be denied coverage. Cathy, my business partner in Diabetes Network, and I were able to buy Blue Cross HMO policies for our business, with no preexisting condition exclusions (and she has type 1 diabetes). Pretty good for a couple of old broads with diabetes.

June and Barbara: We've heard that if a company desperately wants to hire you, you may be able to negotiate a deal with them to pay for your extra coverage during this preexisting condition exclusion period. As Virginia says, though, know what you're getting into before you make any job changes and, of course, make certain all promises are in writing.

But then, what do you do if the insurance change is not by your choice? What if you get caught in a merger or some other corporate upheaval and get laid off? Are you just left hanging out to dry?

Virginia: No, at least not at first. You can take advantage of the government's COBRA plan. Despite the venomous sound of the name, it can be a lifesaver. COBRA stands for Consolidated Omnibus Budget Reconciliation Act, which, I realize, doesn't explain anything about it. What this plan does is give you the right to keep the insurance from your previous employer for up to eighteen months. The bad news is you have to pay the premium yourself. The good news is that if during this eighteen-month period you have an accident or require surgery with a long recuperation period, the insurance company is obligated to keep covering you until the condition is cleared up.

June and Barbara: What if you get laid off and join a new company that has a one-year preexisting condition exclusion? Can you use the COBRA until the preexisting condition period is over?

Virginia: Unfortunately not. The COBRA plan is only for people who have no other health insurance at all. You can't decide to use it just because your new health insurance excludes your diabetes. Supposedly, the Kennedy-Kassebaum Bill protects you from that preexisting condition exclusion, but don't forget the thirty-day rule. Pay the COBRA cost to maintain your coverage so when you get your new insurance you will have continuous coverage.

Medigap and Senior Plans

June and Barbara: A lot of people who are on Medicare buy some kind of so-called Medigap insurance to try to plug up the holes in their Medicare. How does this work—or does it work?

Virginia: The Feds have fine-tuned their regulations on Medigap plans. They fall into closely defined designations, and the company must clearly indicate which plan the customer is getting. Some Medigap plans may cover only the co-payment on Medicare-covered benefits. Other Medigap plans may cover expenses not covered under Medicare. Another option is an HMO that will take your Medicare contract for payment. You see these advertised as "senior plans."

The advantage to senior plans is that you get doctor visits and prescriptions for a small co-payment and no paperwork. The disadvantage is that you probably won't get as much choice about your physician. These programs must run efficiently to make ends meet, and therefore usually offer no-frills care, but that doesn't necessarily mean poor quality. Many times they use nurses for triaging patients in their initial visit, to determine medical priorities, and to make sure they get the correct level of care. Often patients find that they actually prefer getting care from nurses rather than physicians because the nurses do more teaching and spend more time with the patient.

I guess our challenge for the future is how to get Cadillac care for Volkswagen prices. Our health-care system is going to have to become something like a Toyota: efficient, attractive, and moderately priced with excellent quality.

June and Barbara: One thing we can all be sure of is change—and not always for the better. As you said before, every presidential candidate talks about his or her new health plan and then seems to forget about it once in office. Employers are beginning to cut back on health benefits and push more costs onto employees. Some companies (IBM, for instance) even let workers make their own benefits decisions by providing them with medical vouchers to be used on the insurance plan and coverage of their choice. Expect such changes—along with more that nobody's thought of yet—and hope for the best.

7

Diabetes in Children and Young People

Youth Must Be Served—Especially When They Develop Diabetes

BASICALLY, THERE ARE THREE TYPES OF DIABETES THAT occur in children and young people: type 1, type 2, which is here what we're most concerned with, and MODY.

TYPE 1

This is an autoimmune disease. This means the immune system decides for some reason that it hates a particular type of tissue—in this case it's the beta cells in the pancreas that make insulin. When this happens, the body springs into action and starts making antibodies to combat the "enemy" tissue. These antibodies begin killing off the insulin-producing beta cells. Eventually the body is not making enough insulin to keep the blood sugar normal, the blood sugar starts going up, and the result is diabetes.

Often in type 1 there is no family history of diabetes, and these people will require insulin for life.

It is to be hoped that the child or young person is diagnosed with diabetes early on and put on an insulin regimen before going into ketoacidosis. This is a serious condition in which the body starts burning its own fat for fuel and the harmful acid substances formed during the digestion of fat (ketones) are given off.

We now realize this autoimmune type 1 diabetes can occur at any age. I have a number of patients who were diagnosed with type 1 as adults and yet many, like June, spend years believing they were type 2 simply because they were older when diagnosed. (In earlier days legend had it that all adults who developed diabetes were ipso facto type 2.)

TYPE 2

This type has usually been seen in adults, but—unfortunately in recent years—is found increasingly in the young population. The genesis of this disease is insulin resistance, that old devil pancreatic poop-out, and excessive glucose produced by the liver.

We know that diabetes is much more likely to occur in American Indians, African-Americans, Hispanics, and Asians, and now we see that it is occurring at younger and younger ages. It is not unusual now to see children as young as ten with prediabetes and even the real thing diabetes. Interestingly—and distressingly—we now see diabetes occurring ten to fifteen years earlier with each generation.

I have a patient I'm seeing right how who is Hispanic and who is a farmer in a rural area of New Mexico. Henry's wife had already had gastric bypass surgery for obesity. He was seeing me for diabetes management, as he was planning the Lap-Band surgery (see Bariatric Surgery for Obesity in the reference section).

When he came to appointments he often brought with him

his eleven-year-old son, who was significantly overweight. At our last appointment I asked him how he and his wife were working on his son's weight.

He replied, "Well, he really likes his sodas and pizza."

I said, "You know he can't get in the car and go to the store to buy soda. If it isn't in the house he can't drink it."

Henry just laughed.

"Listen, Henry," I told him, "if I were giving my child arsenic, but it was only a little bit each day and he really liked his arsenic, you would try to stop me, wouldn't you?"

Henry just looked at me and said again, "Well, he really likes his sodas."

As we walked to the waiting room, I could see that Henry Jr. already had significant acanthosis nigricans, which indicates that he is on the path to type 2 diabetes. Acanthosis nigricans is a marker for insulin resistance and increased insulin levels. It shows up as darkened pigment and thickened velvety skin around the neck, armpits, and groin. The treatment is weight loss and exercise, which can reduce the pigmentation and the chances of progression to type 2 diabetes.

When a young person develops diabetes, the treatment is difficult because most of the treatments (oral diabetes medications) are not approved for children.

It is fairly well agreed upon by experts that the treatment of choice for adolescent type 2s is metformin and, of course, diet and exercise. Working on weight loss is a real challenge with teenagers because they don't want to be different, and many times the choice of foods available at school and entertainment functions is less than desirable. Some centers actually consider weight-loss surgery for older adolescents who are morbidly obese (50 percent to 100 percent or one hundred pounds above their ideal body weight).

MODY (MATURITY ONSET DIABETES OF YOUTH)

June and Barbara: That used to be considered the same as type 2 diabetes only occurring in young people. Is that still true?

Virginia: No. MODY is a specific genetic defect that leads to high blood glucose levels because of inadequate production of insulin, but not complete insulin deficiency.

The characteristics of MODY include:

1. Early onset of diabetes—usually less than twenty-five years.
2. MODY runs in families through several generations. A parent with MODY has a 50 percent chance of passing on MODY to his or her children. This is called autosomal dominant inheritance—meaning you only need to get the abnormal gene from one parent for you to inherit the disease.
3. People with MODY do not always need insulin treatment and can often be treated with diabetes pills or meal planning alone.
4. People with MODY do not produce enough insulin. This is different from type 2 diabetes, where people frequently produce lots of insulin but don't respond to their insulin.

Here's a little quiz to nail down the concept of these three kinds of diabetes that occur in children and young people:

- A ten-year-old child is diagnosed with diabetes after hospitalization for diabetic ketoacidosis and a blood glucose of 750 mg/dl. Was normal weight but has been losing weight for the last month and is now down twenty pounds. No family history of diabetes except great-grandmother diagnosed with type 2 at seventy-four years.

What type does he have?

ANSWER: Type 1. We can confirm with a blood test called the C-peptide test to see if the child is making insulin and a test (anti-GAD antibody or anti-islet cell antibody test) to see if he is making antibodies to his own beta cells. Treatment will be insulin injections and maybe a pump in a few years.

- A fourteen-year-old girl who is overweight and has a BMI (body mass index) of 42 at a height of 5'4" and a weight of 248 pounds. She has acanthosis nigricans on her neck and armpits and her blood glucose is 180/mg/dl fasting and usually around 250–300 after meals. She has not lost any weight in the last few years.

What type does she have?

ANSWER: Type 2. Turns out most of her family members on both sides have type 2 diabetes and she weighed eleven pounds at birth. Treatment will be to work on weight loss and increasing activity and probably metformin medication.

- A seventeen-year-young man notes that he is urinating more often and is having blurry vision off and on. He is concerned about diabetes because his father was diagnosed at about age twenty and his grandfather was also diagnosed at a young age. His father is not on insulin, but his grandfather does require a small amount. Both are doing well with their diabetes and have no complications.

What type does he have?

ANSWER: In all likelihood, MODY. He will probably respond well to learning how to eat healthy, stay active, and maybe use a sulfonylurea-type medication such as glipizide or small amounts of insulin.

Dietary Considerations for Children and Young People with Type 2 Diabetes

June and Barbara: Virginia, do you think Marion Nestle is as wonderful as we do? We're working on the dietary part of the kids' section and we're going to have to work really hard to keep from making it sound as if it's an application for her sainthood.

Virginia: I LOVE her! I heard her speak . . . and she *is* a saint.

So—in case you aren't familiar with her—just who is this righteous person? Well, she has been called "Nutrition Guru" and "Supermarket Sleuth" and "Obesity Warrior" by fans and less flattering names by food industry spokespersons, to whom she gives conniption fits.

Marion Nestle's credentials include: a doctorate in molecular biology from the University of California, Berkeley; nutrition chair and professor of food studies and public health at New York University; editor of the 1988 Surgeon General's Report; nutrition policy adviser to the Department of Health and Human Services; member of nutrition and science advisory committees to the U.S. Department of Agriculture and the Food and Drug Administration. She is the author of *Food Politics: How the Food Industry Influences Nutrition and Health* and *Safe Food: Bacteria, Biotechnology, and Bioterrorism.* Her latest book is *What to Eat.*

Since this section deals primarily with type 2 children and youths, and since Nestle is passionate about the need for good nutrition and weight loss (when needed) for members of the younger generation, we'll focus here on that group, but actually it applies to all people of all ages, diabetic or not.

In case you haven't noticed, this country is in the throes of an obesity epidemic, which is bringing on a concomitant diabetes epidemic, and Nestle, in materials by and about her on the Internet, gives us a lot of the whys and wherefores and what-you-can-do-about-its there. Following are some of the gleanings of Nestle lore found there.

Food marketers find "insidious ways" to make their products appear healthier. Such foods as cereals and juices, which contain sugar, promote their vitamin content instead and also intimate that eating more of a certain food will increase its nutritional value, when often the reverse is true.

Most yogurt and fruit drinks and many cereals, even those promoted as high fiber or high protein, are loaded with sugars and should be promoted as dessert, not breakfast. Vitamin-enriched sodas are still sodas. Organic Gummi Bears are still candy. Trans-fat-free snack foods are still salty and full of rapidly absorbable carbohydrates.

Nestle emphasizes that although adults may be fair game for marketers, children are not. Marketing to children crosses over the ethical line. Kids cannot distinguish between sales pitches from information unless taught to do so. Food companies spend at least $10 billion annually enticing children to desire food brands and to pester parents to buy them. (These days you can even buy textbooks on how to market to children.) The result: American children consume more than one-third of their daily calories from soft drinks, sweets, salty snacks, and fast food.

Cookie and cereal manufacturers use toys and cartoon figures to reach the younger audience, and soft drink companies also may pay financially strapped schools for the exclusive rights to place vending machines in their cafeterias. (Soft drink machines in schools means the children are essentially drinking liquid candy.)

Nestle believes the worst thing about all of this is that food marketing subverts parental authority by making children believe they are supposed to be eating such foods and they—not their parents—know what is best for them to eat. Today's marketing methods extend beyond television to include Internet games, product placements, character licensing, and word-of-mouth campaigns—in other words, stealth methods likely to be invisible to parents. Controls on marketing may not prevent childhood obesity, but they would make it easier for parents to help children eat more healthfully.

The basic problem is that our country has available in the food supply 3,900 calories for every man, woman, and child—twice as much as the population needs. To make their shareholders happy, food companies have to keep getting people to eat more and/or switch to their products. To do this, they have to change the social environment so it's acceptable for children to drink soft drinks in school—and even have babies drink it in their bottles and for people to snack all day long and to eat food in larger and larger portions.

In the obesity battle it's politically okay to say to exercise more, but never, ever say eat less. This would upset the food industry and cause them to sic their lobbyists onto the representatives to whom they contribute the funds that will enrich their campaign treasuries for the next election. The representatives will then proceed to lean on the appropriate government agencies to make changes the food industry wants.

Nestle, who edited the Surgeon General's Report on Nutrition and Health in 1988, says that what the report actually meant was, "Eat less meat and dairy products and stop eating soft drinks and junk foods and snack foods." But it couldn't say that or—politics as usual—it would get the food industry people in a snit and cause them to label it a "dangerous report" containing un-American statements about eating less meat.

Another problem is that all of a sudden it's okay to eat in bookstores and in libraries and clothing stores, in fact everywhere. Just look around and you'll see it happening. There used to be signs that said don't bring food in here. No more. Temptation abounds.

Nestle also labels supermarkets as danger zones. Her advice for parents: shop the periphery where the fresh fruits and vegetables are. Don't go into the center aisles, the land of processed foods. Don't buy anything with more than five ingredients on the package label. If you can't pronounce the ingredients on the label, don't buy it. Don't buy anything with a cartoon on the package. She adds that markets should be required to shelve healthier products at eye level for easier access. (Lots of luck on that one, Marion.)

In a program at the Potrero Hill (San Francisco area) Parents Organization, Marion Nestle answered the questions that were of greatest concern to those parents and may well be of the greatest concern to you:

PHP: *From unhealthy school lunches to being bombarded by television ads for junk food, it is "tempting" these days for kids to eat the wrong foods. What advice can you give parents to keep their children on track nutritionally?*

NESTLE: I see three problems with junk foods. They are heavily advertised to make kids want them, they are highly processed so they are not as nutritious as "real" foods, and they are loaded with calories which today's kids don't need. Worse, the advertising is designed to make kids think they are supposed to eat these foods, and not the foods that you eat. Kids should be eating foods for grown-ups, just smaller amounts and not heavily salted or sugared.

PHP: *Leading by example, as the saying goes. To what extent do sensible food choices by parents affect what kids will or will not eat?*

NESTLE: How about 100 percent? If you want kids to eat healthily, you have to eat healthily yourself. How's that for a deal?

To sum it up, here's Marion's nutritional mantra for children and adults:

- Eat less.
- Move more.
- Eat fruits and vegetables.
- Don't eat much junk food.
- Eat breakfast every day.

Exercise for Children and Young People with Type 2 Diabetes

"Next to controlling your food intake, getting exercise is probably the best thing you can do to control your diabetes. Unlike medications, exercise is 'all natural' and has no side effects."

—GRETCHEN BECKER
The First Year; Type 2 Diabetes

Exercise is the second major factor in controlling type 2 diabetes, but it is by no means a *secondary* one. It is an incredibly important therapy for all children who have the condition. The basic recommendation is that type 2 children and young people should try to exercise every day for at least thirty minutes—actually an hour would be even better. In what we might now call the good old days, this was automatically taken care of since part of every school day from elementary through high school included some sort of physical education program/exercise period. But in recent years many schools—in order to emphasize academics—have diminished or even eliminated the exercise part of the curriculum. What's really shocking about this anti-exercise tale of woe is that some new high schools are now actually being built without gyms. Put this all together and you have children becoming much more sedentary, and as a result many of these have become obese.

Marion Parrott, M.D., national vice president of clinical affairs of the American Diabetes Association, says that the sharp increase in the number of young adults and children being diagnosed with type 2 diabetes can be attributed to the increasing numbers of obese children, and much of this increase in turn can be attributed to a lack of exercise. Thus the vicious circle spins.

Another part of the problem, Dr. Parrott says, is that many children don't even go out to play after school as they did in days of yore, either because they live in unsafe neighborhoods and/or because their working parents may not be at home to encourage and supervise these physical activities.

To make up for this loss of regular exercise, Dr. Parrot urges the reinstatement of physical education in the schools and the addition of after-school and day programs that include exercise in their regular activities. Parents also need to be urged to plan regular family outings that incorporate physical exertion. That would be good for everyone involved.

And there is another major culprit in this sedentary/obesity/ type 2 diabetes equation. Read on.

Television

A few years ago while on a trip to Turkey, we kept noticing shops featuring jewelry and plaques with a representation of a blue eye. We asked what it was and were told that it was to ward off the evil eye and bring good luck. Ever-superstitious Barbara, feeling we needed all the good luck we could get, picked up a little group of evil eye repellants on a chain, which she later hung on a lamp overlooking our computer workstation. It didn't work perfectly, since June had her stroke three years later.

But even so, we don't feel you should ignore the evil eye that you have right there in your home and the damage it can do to all the members of your household—especially to any type 2 young people who may reside there. We're referring to the flickering evil eye of that old devil TV.

Actually, making time for exercise by cutting down TV watching is one of the best type 2 diabetes therapies imaginable. A *New York Times* article told of a study by psychologist Robert Klesges of Memphis State University. He discovered that when children watch television, "they lapse into a deeply relaxed almost semiconscious state somewhere between resting and sleeping." This lowers their metabolic rate so that these children burn fewer calories watching TV than they would if they sat still doing nothing, and almost as few as if they were sleeping. This may well contribute to the epidemic of obesity and type 2 diabetes in children and young people.

Dr. Klesges believes that this TV-induced drop in metabolic rate could be a major contributor to the obesity epidemic in this country. In other words, it's the opposite of Covert Bailey's exercise-induced revving up of the metabolism (see page 110). So cut down on TV-watching for the whole family. It will prevent softening of the body as well as softening of the brain.

P.S. If you happen to be traveling in Turkey or Greece, you might pick up something decorated with an evil eye to put on your TV to remind you to turn it off—or, better still, to not turn it on. If you don't have any such trips on the offing, you can always look up Evil Eye Jewelry on the Internet and find something to order there. (As we keep telling you, you really need to get on the Internet.)

Too Little Sleep

Yes, obesity can bring out diabetes and, yes, America's children seem to be in the throes of an obesity epidemic. Of course, many Americans of all ages have a weight problem. We have friends who travel overseas frequently and one of their pastimes while there is to stroll along a street in a foreign city and point out obese people and say to each other (sotto voce, of course), "American. American. American."

But that's another equally depressing story. What we're concerned with here are the overweight, going-on-obese American children. We feel if we can get them while they're young and change them, we'll have them for life—and a longer and healthier life that will be.

Marion Nestle has given us the dietary part of the children's health and weight control equation, but there is another aspect to consider: sleep. Sleep? Yes. More and more studies from New Zealand to Scotland to Michigan are giving us the surprising revelation that children who sleep too little are at risk for overweight and obesity.

A New Zealand study of 519 seven-year-olds revealed that those who slept less than nine hours a night could be overweight and/or obese.

A larger (9,000 children) and longer (birth to seven years) study in Scotland by Dr. John Reilly of the University of Glasgow reinforced the idea of not getting enough sleep as a factor in childhood obesity. Among the other contributing factors, he included parental influence of transmitted genes (which can't be helped) and the food favored at the family dinner table. (Hail, Marion!)

In a new study from the University of Michigan's Center for Human Growth and Development the researchers came to believe that the weight gain caused by lack of sleep could be due to several factors, including:

- Tired children have less energy and are less likely to play and exercise during the day than well-rested kids are.
- Children may be more likely to eat larger amounts of junk food when they are irritable or moody because of lack of sleep.
- A lack of sleep can have a strong effect on important hormones that affect fat storage, appetite, and glucose metabolism.
- If you find the nine-hour sleep requirement for children a little hard to swallow, now hear this: the National Sleep Foundation's opinion is that young children in elementary school should be getting ten to twelve hours of quality sleep per night.

And finally, to end on a paradoxical note, the Palo Alto Medical Foundation's Community Health Resource Center newsletter informs us that children who are overtired from lack of sleep will often have greater difficulty falling asleep than children who are well rested.

Diabetes in Children and Young People: A Summing Up

KPCC, our local public radio station in Pasadena, had on its program *AirTalk* a one-hour feature on childhood diabetes featuring such luminaries as Dr. Francine Kaufman, head of the Center for Diabetes, Endocrinology, and Metabolism at Children's Hospital Los Angeles and the president of the Los Angeles Unified School District, Marlene Cantor.

The discussion—which included calls from listeners—covered such topics as changes in the food and drink policies in schools. First they banned sodas, then went on to banning all junk food. Next they improved the cafeteria environment with comfortable chairs and inviting colors and then laid out the foods attractively so students could see and choose what they wanted. (They said what a joy it was to see kids piling their plates with choices from the salad bar and the fruit bar.) They're now looking forward to a change from white rice to brown.

They discussed the possibility of putting farmers' markets on high school campuses to perk up neighborhood eating and, not incidentally, perk up the school coffers to make up for the loss of the soda subsidy.

In lower-income areas, where there were few markets featuring produce, they suggested trying to get liquor stores (of which there was a plethora) to stock a selection of fruits and vegetables so the less affluent will have easier access to healthy foods.

Of course they emphasized wanting parents to be brought into play—literally and figuratively—with family outings that include exercise. And, since many families must out of necessity eat often in fast-food places, they could be encouraged to try to get the fast-food places to put nutritional information on their labels so the family members will know what they're eating. (Of course, they said the fast-food industry is resisting this change, for obvious reasons.)

Being realists, the discussion group recognized that all the changes they were aiming for couldn't happen overnight. They suggested starting with small changes, then gradually moving on to the major ones that everyone wanted.

Since this program had knowledgeable participants, all of whom had many important ideas to contribute, you really should hear the whole shebang. Fortunately, you can. KPCC has made it possible for you to order a CD copy of the *AirTalk* segment on "Diabetes in Children" by calling (1-626-585-7000) or faxing (1-626-585-7916) the station. Or you can listen to the segment by going on to the Web site www.kpcc.org; click on *AirTalk* and search for the date, May 25, 2007.

8

Taking the Risk
Out of Risk Factors

WE LONG AGO DECIDED THAT IF WE RULED THE WORLD WE'D INSTI-
tute a new law. If you had one disease, that would be it. For example,
if you developed diabetes, that's all you get. No more health problems
for you! Well, as you may have noticed, despite our obvious qualifica-
tions for the job, we weren't appointed world rulers. Therefore, all we
can do is to try to make the best of the situation. We urge you to be
alert to the risk factors for other health problems that people with di-
abetes are sometimes subject to, and to do everything in your power
to avoid them. Then, if, despite all of our mutual best efforts, another
physical problem raises its ugly head, we must learn the best ways
and means of handling the situation.

—June and Barbara

Not the Only Game in Town

Ever since June was diagnosed with diabetes way back in 1967 and we started researching and writing about it, diabetes has totally occupied our hearts and minds. It was all diabetes, all the time, 24/7, awake or asleep. As a result, when anything went awry with June's health, we always attributed it to diabetes, and if truth be told, it almost always was.

And yet as the years went by, we learned the hard way that although diabetes occupies center stage in our lives, *it is not the only health game in town*. Along with the other ailments and medical problems to which all of humankind is susceptible, people with diabetes need to pay particular attention to the two biggies— major risk factors associated with diabetes—heart attacks and strokes. We'll discuss these two here and, since there are some minor (only minor in the sense of being somewhat less common) diabetes risk factors, we'll also cover one of those, glaucoma, that June, whom we affectionately call "the woman who has everything," also experienced.

Heart Attack and Cardiac Arrest

If you're looking for something to worry about and take serious measures to prevent, and to recognize the symptoms if it happens, heart attacks are the number one candidate, since they are the number one health problem.

All of the associations involved with the heart attacks say the same thing. It is generally not what they like to call a "movie" heart attack when the person having it dramatically clutches his or her chest and falls to the ground. Actually, for the most part, heart attacks are much more subtle than this. Often you don't even know you're having one—you know *something* is wrong, but you don't know what. The attack can start slowly with nothing more than a mild pain or uncomfortable feeling which may come and go. Unfortunately, this may cause the person having the attack to think it's nothing and just ignore it. Of course, this is the worst thing you can do, whether it's you who is having these vague feelings or a family member or friend. *Immediately* call the paramedics (911). Fast action is vital in a heart attack situation. Don't let embarrassment of It's-probably-nothing-I-don't-want-to-create-a-scene keep you from the care you may need to save your life or the life of another. If it turns out it really *is* nothing, just celebrate the happy situation and go about your business.

There are many warning signs of a heart attack:

1. An uncomfortable feeling of pressure or pain or fullness in the center of the chest that lasts longer than a few minutes. It may go away and then come back.
2. A feeling of discomfort in the upper body. It could be in one or both arms, the back, neck, jaw, or even in the stomach.
3. Shortness of breath sometimes along with discomfort in the chest, or it could occur before the chest discomfort.
4. Other miscellaneous symptoms, which could include nausea, breaking out in a sweat, light-headedness, or dizziness.

Strangely enough, even if you've had one heart attack and think you'd recognize it if you have another, that's not necessarily so because the next heart attack could have totally different symptoms.

The Sooner, the Better

The reason we keep emphasizing fast action is because quickly administered artery-opening drugs (such as so-called "clot busters") prevent or limit the damage to the heart.

Other Risk Factors

Although your diabetes is the risk factor we're emphasizing here, it's not the only one you may be subjected to, so be alert to the following and avoid them when possible:

1. Smoking.
2. Age, alas, this is not something we can do much about; 83 percent of the people who die from heart disease are sixty-five or older.
3. High cholesterol.
4. High blood pressure.
5. A family history of heart attacks.
6. Your race. You are at greater risk if you are African-American, Hispanic American, American Indian, or Hawaiian.
7. Hardening of the arteries.
8. Lack of exercise.
9. Stress.
10. Obesity.
11. Gender. More males have heart attacks than women, but heart disease is the leading cause of death for American women.

Heart Attacks in Women

There's some good news and bad news. Women usually are ten years older than men when they have a heart attack, but they are more likely to have other conditions along with it such as, you guessed it, diabetes, high blood pressure, and congestive heart failure. As with all heart attacks, a speedy response is of the essence for a good outcome.

Strokes

Considering our laser-beam focus on diabetes, it's not surprising that one day when we were getting ready to go to a play and June started slurring her speech and generally acting peculiar, I immediately thought, "uh-oh, I guess she has low blood sugar." But when we took it, it turned out to be perfectly normal, and before long, June appeared to be normal again, too.

What must have happened, we reasoned (make that "rationalized"), was that she had *had* low blood sugar, but since we didn't do anything early on to correct it, the good old reliable liver kicked out some sugar to take care of the situation. That's why the test didn't show she had low blood sugar.

After that was cleared up, we went off to the play and thought no more about it. But a few months later June had another "incident." This one was more dramatic and more serious. Not only did she have trouble speaking as before, but her right leg was too weak for her to stand on. This was like no low blood sugar she'd ever experienced. We decided it was paramedic time.

Once in the emergency room she began to get better. The neurologist checked her out with the finger test (how many fingers do you see?) and talked to her ascertaining that her speech was okay. I wanted to take her home, but they wanted to keep her overnight. (Hospital rule: once you're taken to the hospital, they usually make you stay overnight "just to be sure." If you have good insurance, they *always* make you stay overnight.)

Not to keep you in suspense, what June had was what is known as a TIA—a transient ischemic attack. This is sometimes called a "mini stroke" or a "warning stroke." This is usually very brief and not permanently damaging. Unlike a full-blown stroke, a TIA is a temporary interruption of blood flow to the brain when little bits of foreign matter lodge in small blood vessels there. When this interrupts the flow of blood to an area of the brain, that area stops functioning until the bits of vascular rubble are dissolved. These episodes last from minutes to hours, with full recovery within twenty-four hours. They should not, however, be ignored: in the United States, more than one-third of individuals who experience a TIA will have the real thing within five years.

June was told to take a daily baby aspirin, and life returned to normal. We even took a trip to Amsterdam and Paris. But upon our return and after celebrating June's birthday with friends the following morning, June experienced major constipation. She had had this condition before, sometimes requiring intervention in a proctologist's office. But over the years she got by with glycerin suppositories and, in later stages, Fleet enemas. But this time the impaction was so great that neither the water nor the oil variety worked its customary magic. Finally, after an hour of "straining at stool," as they say in medical talk, the impaction finally broke. But that was not all that broke. June suddenly felt the symptoms of a real stroke. She had the slurred speech again, and a weakness on her right side. I immediately took her to the hospital, but by the time we got there she couldn't walk and had to be lifted into a wheelchair and carted into the ER. What she had was a hemorrhagic stroke, which happens when a damaged or diseased blood vessel in the brain ruptures, resulting in bleeding in the brain. For obvious reasons, this is colloquially known as a "bleeder." This kind of stroke is relatively rare—only 12 per cent of all strokes are of this type.

If you want to know more about June's strokes and the aftermaths, we wrote a book about them: *The Stroke Book: A Guide to Life After Stroke for Survivors and Those Who Care for Them.* But we wanted to tell you here about June's experience because we now have another mission in life along with helping people learn to live long and happily with diabetes. This secondary mission is to spread the word about something that you are seldom if ever told about—the very serious danger of straining at stool. The doctors that oversaw June's hospital stay considered our idea that constipation and concomitant straining at stool could have caused the stroke ludicrous—just another loony theory from an ignorant layperson.

But as is our habit, we didn't give up pursuing this idea, and the higher up we went on the medical food chain, the more substantiation we received. First, our gynecologist said, "Of course that could have caused it. The pressure on the blood vessels from straining at stool is tremendous. As a matter of fact, even a hearty sneeze can cause a break in a blood vessel."

Our beloved diabetes oracle, Virginia, echoed his sentiments: "Yes, certainly straining at stool can cause increased intracranial and intrathoracic pressure. That's why they give post-MI [myocardial infarction] patients stool softeners in the ICU. It is also why we recommend folks with diabetes don't engage in lifting heavy weights, because of the increased blood pressure when they strain to lift heavy weights."

So there you have it. Tell your family and friends—shucks, even tell your enemies, if you have any.

Alzheimer's

This is not usually counted among the most common diabetes risk factors, but times they are a-changing. As it's more prevalent among the general population, Alzheimer's is becoming a growing diabetes risk factor as well. A study in the *Archives of Neurology* indicates that diabetics have a 65 percent higher risk of developing Alzheimer's than the average person.

Another six-year study of 824 members of religious orders revealed that 151 of those in the study developed Alzheimer's and of those 31 had diabetes. The conclusion was a 65 percent (there's that magic number again!) increase in the risk of developing Alzheimer's among people who are diabetic.

Researchers have long known that people with diabetes have a greater risk of developing Alzheimer's and other forms of dementia, but they haven't known why. With the incidence of it growing, though, they're starting to get serious about finding out the reason. A new joint study between researchers in Cologne, Germany, and Boston's Joslin Diabetes Center suggests that insulin resistance in brain cells can cause biochemical changes similar to those found in patients with Alzheimer's.

Research at the Joslin Diabetes Center also has come to the realization that insulin receptors are present in all tissues of the body, including the brain, and they may affect the function of these tissues.

All this research is just in the beginning stages. They have yet to figure out how insulin resistance in the brain's neurons interacting with other genetic and biochemical abnormalities leads to Alzheimer's and, although theories abound (including one that diabetes might cause an excess amount of glucose in the brain, which damages brain cells), the process that links Alzheimer's disease to diabetes remains unclear.

One particularly fascinating theory is that Alzheimer's might actually be a neuroendocrine disorder. This theory is not new (it was kicked around—and dropped—twenty years ago), but it was revisited in 2005 by Suzanne de la Monte, a neuropathologist at Brown University Medical School. In her research, she made two discoveries that indicated that the brain makes its own insulin and Alzheimer's depletes that insulin resulting in a disease process she termed type 3 diabetes.

This theory is understandably controversial in the diabetes community where the prevailing belief is that Alzheimer's is a complication of diabetes and not a unique form of the disease. "Nevertheless," as Dr. Sue Kirkman, vice president of clinical affairs for the American Diabetes Association, says, "this is primarily a semantic argument." And Dr. de la Monte sees the semantic splitting of hairs as a good thing because "people are arguing about small parts of the bigger story," she says. "At the end of the day, these conversations will help us to better understand both diabetes and Alzheimer's disease."

So until the Alzheimer's/diabetes dust settles, what's a conscientious diabetic to do? As is often the case, our Mayo Clinic friends have the answer. In their *Tools for Healthier Living* newsletter they say that you can counter insulin resistance, which may lead to Alzheimer's, through modest weight loss (if you are overweight, lose 5 percent of your body weight) and exercising thirty minutes most days of the week.

In addition to possibly reducing your risk of Alzheimer's, these lifestyle changes will also help protect you from heart attacks and strokes. In other words, you get three risk factor removals for the price of one. What a bargain!

Glaucoma

A CAUTIONARY TALE OF AN ACUTE GLAUCOMA INCIDENT

We were always warned about the risk of diabetic retinopathy and told how to prevent it with careful blood sugar control. But, as Judith Curtis says in her book *Living with Diabetic Complications*: "people with diabetes are especially prone to this eye disease (glaucoma) that mainly strikes people over forty. Glaucoma usually occurs without symptoms and can only be detected by an ophthalmologist through a series of tests." That's why it is known as "the silent thief of vision." We present this personal experience in the belief that if it saves the sight in even one eye of one person, it will be well worth adding to this book.

Just as we were in the throes of finishing up a book, something unexpected happened. June has always taken meticulous care of her blood sugar (6 to 8 blood sugars a day, injecting five times a day with occasional supplements when needed). The main reason she's been so careful is that, as a college librarian and writer, her eyes are her most precious commodity. She feels no effort is too great to protect them from the demon retinopathy. Because of all this care and the fact that she had no known complications after thirty-five years of diabetes, June felt she had everything under control in the eye department. Oh, yes, she has had "a touch of glaucoma" for the previous five years, but no big deal. It was well controlled with Timoptic drops. Nothing to worry about.

When her regular ophthalmologist retired, she started with a new one who wisely decided to give her a thorough examination. One thing the new doctor noticed in the iris of June's right eye was a lesion. The dictionary translates this medical talk as "a localized abnormal structural change." She thought there was a chance that it could be a melanoma—a small malignant tumor. After we sweated through tests, it turned out to be only a blood vessel. We heaved mighty sighs of relief, and the doctor decided not to do anything about it unless it got worse, in which case she'd zap it with a laser.

It did get worse: it started bleeding, causing June's vision to get foggy, and the doctor did zap. But still it continued to bleed, in fact more so. And every time it bled, June had three or four hours of foggy vision in that eye.

June was sent to the Doris Stein Eye Research Center at the University of California, Los Angeles, for an ultrasound to see what was going on. They suggested more laser treatments until the lesion closed up (warning that care should be exercised lest the eye get fried). More laser treatments ensued. The iris continued to bleed. Back to UCLA, where they used up half a day and untold dollars making tests. After a conference with the big gun doctors there, it was decided that June should sleep with six inches of books beneath the head part of her mattress, keep a diary of her eye problems, and come back in three months. In the letter to June's doctor it was said that the "feeder vessel" had actually been closed by the laser treatments, but there was a "cystic space" (a closed cavity or sac) from whence blood was still draining.

Feeling that everything was on track, we relaxed and waited for the cystic space to drain. A week later at bedtime, June's eye was bleeding and her vision was foggy. Then suddenly she awoke at 2:30 a.m. with an excruciating pain in her eye, nausea, and no vision at all in her right eye. As soon as the office opened, we called for permission and raced June over to the Valley Eye Center, home of her ophthalmologist, where a doctor measured June's eye pressure. It was 80! (Normal is under 20, so you might say this was the crisis equivalent to a 500 blood sugar in diabetes.)

They got to work trying to bring the pressure down with a smorgasbord of eye drops. After spending all morning trying to lower the pressure to no avail, they decided to take June over to the Valley Presbyterian Hospital for a YAG laser treatment to make channels to let out the blood that was causing the pressure buildup. (Since the laser schedule was full, they had to fit her in during the lunch hour when the laser center was normally closed. It was that much of an emergency.)

Back to the Valley Eye Center to measure the pressure every forty-five minutes to see if they could get it low enough to suspend the treatments and let her go home. June was still in great pain during all this, and the nausea was extreme. She was continuously and profusely vomiting into a selection of wastebaskets, which fortunately were lined with plastic. Finally at about 4:00 p.m. (she'd been there since 8:00 a.m.) they decided that while her eye pressure certainly wasn't normal, it was at least down to a little over 40, so they let her go home armed with five different medications and a treatment schedule.

Saturday dawned and June still was feeling far from perfect. But her super conscientious doctor (who lives way down in Manhattan Beach, about forty minutes away) wanted to meet her at the office to take another pressure measurement. This we gladly did, and were delighted to learn the pressure was below 20. But June still couldn't see anything out of her right eye. It was as if a light-colored blind had been pulled down over it. The doctor explained that there was a blood clot over her pupil that was blocking her vision. The doctor said that it could take as long as two weeks for the clot to go away, and if it didn't happen by then, they'd have to give her a special treatment at UCLA with a new laser-type instrument they had just acquired.

Home again to a new wrinkle—this time one related to diabetes. One of the medications contained cortisone. When this was given to her at the eye clinic, we bleated that cortisone would really mess up her blood sugar. They patiently explained that there was so little of it and it was so far away (far away from where?) that it wouldn't affect her blood sugar, especially if she pressed the corner of her eye for two minutes after each time she used the eye drops that contained cortisone. That way it wouldn't get into her system. Although she followed the instructions, her blood sugar shot up to 185 and no matter how she kept increasing her insulin, it stayed in that vicinity.

The doctor who called frequently (we think June may have been her most challenging case) told June she could cut back on the cortisone drops to two a day instead of four. Noncompliant

June cut back to zero drops a day until she got her blood sugar back in control.

A terrifying aside: When June was having her first crisis examination on the infamous Friday, Barbara sat in the office reading the available eye-problem brochures, one of which was on glaucoma. It contained a section on acute glaucoma, which described June's exact symptoms: pain, nausea, and lack of vision. Then in boldface it said: "It develops quickly and can cause blindness in twenty-four hours," and went on to add: "Emergency treatment should be sought immediately." Naturally, Barbara didn't reveal this bit of intelligence to June, but she was on the verge of hyperventilating and passing out after reading it. Luckily, she held it off—that was all we needed.

June went back to UCLA for the special laser treatment, which did no good at all. So she had to go back the following day for a new treatment (it had to be done within twenty-four hours—time was of the essence!). At that time the medication TPA (known in the trade as "the clot buster") was injected into the clot in her pupil to try to break it up. The doctor there said this was not a standard use of the drug, and there was only a fifty-fifty chance that it would work, but at least it would do no harm. Well, it did some harm in that it made the eye extremely painful and caused it to swell shut, but made absolutely no improvement in the total lack of vision in her right eye. When we reported the situation to the doctor who had done the injection, he insisted that we go somewhere immediately to get the pressure measured. Luckily, we were able to slip into the Valley Eye Center just before closing and, even more luckily, we got the doctor who had done the laser treatment on June's eye on that infamous Friday. She found the pressure was 34, which wasn't ideal but not in the danger zone.

That night we reached the nadir of discouragement since June still couldn't see out of her right eye, and we thought that surgery to remove the clot was now the only option—that's what the doctor had said. And who knew if that could work?

The following morning, a strange thing happened. When June looked through her right eye she could dimly see the outline of the venetian blind slats. Maybe something was happening! The UCLA doctor, who also has an office in the Valley, called June to see when she could come to his Valley office so he could meet her there to check the pressure again. When he looked into the eye—oh, happy day!—he discovered that the medication had worked, the clot was gone, and the pupil was again functioning. The reason June couldn't see any better than she did was that all the blood cells from the clot were still floating around—and (sigh!) the pressure was up to 50. The doctor gave her a local anesthetic, inserted a needle, and sucked out blood. The pressure immediately dropped down to 9. June didn't see much better because there was still so much blood on the scene.

But that night while we were watching television, June suddenly announced, "I can see the screen!" and so she could. Our elation knew no bounds, and we both slept better that night than we had for over a week.

Our joy was somewhat tempered by the fact that she had a lot more trouble seeing in the glare of daylight than she did in the half light of television, but she had no pain. She still had a touch of nausea, however, and thought that might indicate that the pressure was again building. But when she checked in with the doctor, as he had requested, he believed that she was right on track and that soon the residual blood cells would be dissipated and the fogginess would be gone. June had an appointment with her Valley doctor on the following Wednesday, and we all hoped that things would be pretty much back to normal by then.

They weren't. She still had the foggy, foggy eye. But when the doctor did a careful, in-depth examination of the eye, she found that the fogginess was, indeed, due to the itinerant red blood cells and that they would surely clear up in time. As June said, "the prescription is patience," plus three of the original five medications. But the best news of all was that the examination revealed that there was no damage to the optic nerve (this is what causes blindness in acute glaucoma attacks), no rubeosis (a condition characterized by a new formation of vessels and connective tissue on the surface of the iris, frequently seen in people with diabetes, which gives rise to severe intractable glaucoma), and no trace of retinopathy. All that meticulous blood sugar maintenance had paid off!

Although June thought her eyesight hadn't improved, a week later a test revealed that she was seeing two lines better on the eye chart than on the previous visit. The doctor assured her that it would keep improving, scheduled the next appointment for three to four weeks later, and cut back on the medications. Crisis past! So this story has a very happy ending.

We've told you this tale not to give you something to worry about, but to give you something to be careful of. Make those regular visits to your ophthalmologist that Virginia put in her commandments, and during the examinations that she advises, be sure to have checks for glaucoma. If it turns out you have it, see your ophthalmologist at least three times a year for regular checks of the pressure. (More frequent visits may be necessary to be certain that the medications remain effective.) And if you ever, ever have those three symptoms of acute glaucoma—pain in the eye, blurred or lack of vision, and nausea—act immediately. Remember that it is an emergency situation. But also remember that if an emergency should occur and the appropriate steps are taken, you, too, can have a bad story with a very happy ending.

(With indescribable appreciation to June's Sainted Sight Savers, all of whom treated her with total selflessness and the highest professional excellence: Doreen T. Fazio, M.D., and Kay L. Park, M.D., of the Valley Eye Center in Van Nuys, California, and Robert E. Engstrom Jr., M.D., of the Doris Stein Eye Research Center, University of California, Los Angeles.)

The ACCORD Study: What You Need to Know

It is a much more complicated issue than was described by *The New York Times*, which simplified the issue to: "major federal study of more than 10,000 middle-aged and older people with type 2 diabetes has found that lowering blood sugar actually increased their risk of death, researchers reported Wednesday." As Kelly Close from Close Concerns describes the situation, science has thrown us a curve ball. She summarizes the issues beautifully in her newsletter:

> Progress in diabetes, it seems, rarely moves in a linear fashion. If last month was a step forward, this month was two separate steps backward. Let's review them in order:
>
> First, *The New England Journal of Medicine* reported that intensive insulin therapy in the ICU may be bad for patients because of increased hypoglycemia. The trial, which compared intensive and conventional insulin therapy in the ICU, was halted due to a potentially dangerous increase in hypoglycemia in patients receiving intensive insulin regimens. Second, preliminary results of the ACCORD trial were disclosed—which, in our view, have left patients and providers with difficult questions about optimal care. In this 10,000-patient study, the intensive treatment arm was halted due to increased mortality in the conventional treatment arm.
>
> In both of these trials, it seems that science has

thrown the diabetes community a curveball. These findings raise doubts about the most important assumptions in diabetes care, and offer the message that intensive glucose control is inherently dangerous for diabetes patients.

I can highly recommend Kelly's newsletter, *Diatribe*. For subscription information, go to www.diatribe.us.

Here's what we know so far about these research studies:

The ADVANCE study randomly assigned 11,140 patients with type 2 diabetes to either standard glucose control or intensive glucose control, defined as the use of gliclazide (similar to glipizide and glyburide in the United States) plus other drugs as required to achieve an A1C of 6.5 percent or less. The study was designed to measure death from cardiovascular causes, nonfatal cardiovascular events, or heart attack, stroke, or major microvascular events such as new cases or worsening of eye or kidney disease. After an average of five years of follow-up, the average A1C level was lower in the intensive-control group (6.5 percent) than in the standard-control group (7.3 percent). The conclusions were that a strategy of intensive glucose control, involving a sulfonylurea and other drugs as required, resulted in a 21 percent reduction in nephropathy (kidney disease) but no change in cardiovascular events.

The ACCORD study was designed to look at many factors that could be modified to reduce cardiovascular disease. It randomly assigned 10,251 patients (average age, 62.2 years) with an average A1C of 8.1 percent to receive either intensive therapy or standard therapy. Of these patients, 38 percent were women, and 35 percent had undergone a previous cardiovascular event. The finding of higher mortality in the intensive-therapy group led to a discontinuation of intensive therapy after 3.5 years of follow-up.

After one year, the intensive group achieved an average A1C of 6.4 percent and the standard therapy group achieved an A1C of 7.5 percent. As compared with standard therapy, the use of intensive therapy to target normal A1C levels for 3.5 years increased mortality by 20 percent and did not significantly reduce major cardiovascular events. These results took all of us by surprise. A thorough analysis of all therapies and patient groups did not identify a particular medication or combination of medications or hypoglycemic or other single event that could explain these results. It seems that this unexpected outcome was due to a therapy approach using many different medications in combination to get a rapid lowering of glucose to near normal levels in a group of people who were at high rish for heart disease (more than one-third had previous cardiovascular event such as heart attack or stroke). Patients in the intensive-therapy group who did not have a history of a cardiovascular event or whose baseline A1C level was below 8 percent had significantly fewer fatal and nonfatal cardiovascular events than did patients at higher risk. These findings suggest that intensive therapy was beneficial at least in this small group. Whether achieving glucose targets below 7 percent will be good for all patients with type 2 diabetes and a low risk of cardiovascular disease remains another unanswered question. Both studies used statin-type drugs (Lipitor) and blood pressure medications to achieve good control of cholesterol and blood pressure. We also noted that both groups had better mortality rates than the general population did.

What do we make of these two trials? The good news, AD-VANCE showed us again that improving glucose control helps reduce microvascular problems such as kidney disease. Both studies failed to show improvement in cardiovascular disease, at least in 3– to 5-year studies, and, in fact, for some people, trying to get below

6.5 percent A1C could be harmful. Studies will continue to follow these patients, and over time we may see different results. In the EDICT study, the continuation of the DCCT study, it took more than ten years to see an improvement in cardiovascular events in the intensive group, but they did not have A1C levels as low as with ACCORD. So, for now, talk to your health-care professional about what your goals should be. If you are new to diabetes and don't have cardiovascular problems, you can probably benefit from getting close to normal as long as you don't have too much low glucose. If you have had diabetes for more than eight or ten years and suffer from heart problems, you should probably shoot for a gradual reduction to a 7 percent A1C.

9

Two Little Afterwords

At My Age, Why Should I Bother?

Now that we've come to the end of the questions about type 2 diabetes, we're left with just one question—the one we've heard more than any other from people who are diagnosed with diabetes in their adult years:

- At my age, why should I bother making all these changes?
- At my age, why should I start a whole new way of eating? I like the way I've always eaten.
- At my age, why should I start exercising? I've never liked exercise. I didn't like it when I was younger and I like it even less now.
- At my age, why should I try to lose weight? It's not easy—I should know because I've tried to do it dozens of times, and the weight never stays off anyway.

- At my age, why should I stick my fingers and take all those blood sugars? It doesn't feel good and it's expensive.
- What possible good can doing all these things do me at my age?

We agree. If you're an oldie, you definitely shouldn't bother. It's a waste of time and it probably won't do you any good at all. Your next question might logically be, at exactly what age do you become an oldie?

That's not an easy one to answer. We've seen oldies who were in their twenties and thirties, and we've seen people in their nineties who were definitely not oldies. June started using the term "oldie" when she herself was in her sixties, and she often used it in reference to people who were much younger than herself. She's always pointing out oldies doing such things as driving about 40 miles per hour in the fast lane of the freeway or unconsciously and inconsiderately blocking supermarket aisles with their shopping carts.

One of her favorite experiences occurred back when we were running the SugarFree Center. June answered the phone one day. It was a woman calling to cancel her appointment to learn how to use a meter. The reason she gave for canceling was, "You see, I'm sixty years old." June, who was sixty-four at the time, mused to herself, "What does being sixty have to do with canceling an appointment? . . . Oh well, I guess she's just an oldie."

When pressed to sum up exactly what an oldie is, June says it's a person who has given up on himself or herself. As we said before, that can happen at any age. But it's true that the older you get the greater the temptation to fall victim to the oldie syndrome.

If you want to see whether you are developing the "condition," try taking the following test:

1. Do you use your age as an excuse for getting out of doing things?
2. Do you expect others to do special things for you? That is to say, do you have an "I need to be taken care of" turn of mind?
3. Even if you're financially well off and secure, do you feel poor and hesitate to spend money on yourself for things that would make you healthier and happier?
4. Do you use your age as an excuse—even if it's just to yourself—for being unhappy?
5. Do you generally resist trying new things?
6. Do you usually try to avoid responsibility?
7. If you're not retired yet, do you look forward to retirement as a time when you can "just do nothing"? If you are retired, do you spend most of your time "just doing nothing"?
8. Do you feel the best part of your life is over?
9. Do you focus on what you can't do rather than on what you can do?
10. Do you feel you're too old and that your mind doesn't work well enough now to try to work new electronic or technological devices—for example, the automatic teller machine at the bank, a computer, a VCR, or, most significantly, a blood sugar meter?
11. Do you often feel sorry for yourself?
12. Do you think more about the past than about the present and future?
13. Do you have a lot of regrets?
14. Do you have more things that you dread than things that you look forward to?
15. Do you often find yourself saying—or even thinking—such phrases as "What's the use?" or "It's just not worth the effort"?
16. Do you feel that you're too old to do most of the things you'd really like to do?

17. Do you primarily think of yourself and your needs rather than others and their needs?

Count how many yes answers you have. As you may have suspected, this quiz is like one of those "Are you an alcoholic?" quizzes in which even one yes answer is cause for concern. If you answered yes to one or more questions, you either are an oldie or are well on the way to becoming one.

But all is not lost. You don't have to be an oldie. Diabetes may be just the wake-up call you need to push you off the oldie track. We both practice oldie prevention with every fiber of our beings, and it must be working at least a little. A few years ago after a talk we gave in Salt Lake City, a woman came up to us and said, "I hope you'll take this in the right way, but from reading your books, I'd think you're a lot younger than you really are." We did take it in the right way—except that she was a little wrong in her assessment. Our real ages are not necessarily the ones that our birth certificates would indicate—and neither is yours. We recently heard a saying attributed to the baseball player/philosopher Satchel Paige: "How old would you be if you didn't know how old you were?" Ponder that one a minute. And then possibly experience a little shudder of horror at the possibility that if you didn't know how old you were, you might be a decade or two older from the way you're conducting your life.

A famous yachtsman once said: "Somewhere in the corner of your heart, you're always twenty-two years old." Now's the time to find that corner and expand it until it occupies your whole heart. Because it still is possible for you to be twenty-two years old in all the ways that really count, and one of the most important is feeling that many wonderful moments lie ahead, which will motivate you to take good care of yourself so you can enjoy them to the fullest.

At your age—whatever that age may be—it is worth the bother and, more important, you're worth the bother.

—*June and Barbara*

The Diabetes Gospel According to Virginia Valentine

One of the rules for giving a speech is "Tell them what you're going to tell them. Tell them. Then tell them what you told them." The same rule holds true for a book. We've done the first two and now we'll end by having Virginia tell you the most important part of what she's already told you. She's doing this in the form of a loving valentine: "The Fifteen Commandments for Living Well with Diabetes." (She says this means that it's 50 percent more difficult to have diabetes than to be a good Christian or Jew.) We think you should make a copy of this and put it on your refrigerator, bathroom mirror, or some other place where you'll see it frequently.

VIRGINIA'S FIFTEEN COMMANDMENTS
FOR LIVING WELL WITH DIABETES

1. Thou shalt find a doctor and diabetes educator who understand that type 2 diabetes is not a character flaw and who will work with thee to achieve normal range blood sugar goals, and thou shalt honor them.
2. Thou shalt visit thy doctor and diabetes educator every three months for monitoring of thy diabetes with an A1C test and checking for possible complications.
3. Thou shalt work with the dietitian to design a livable, yet healthy diet (high-fiber, low-fat) that includes goodies now and then so thou won't covet gooey sweets and pig out.
4. Thou shalt have thy blood pressure and cholesterol and triglycerides monitored every year and follow the diet and

medication regimen to get them in the normal range. Also, ask thy doctor if thou should be taking a baby aspirin every day to lower thy risk of heart attack.

5. Thou shalt have thy urine checked for microalbuminuria (microscopic levels of protein) every year and have any urinary tract or bladder infections treated immediately.

6. Thou shalt see thy ophthalmologist at least annually for a dilated eye exam (see "A Cautionary Tale of an Acute Glaucoma Incident").

7. Thou shalt care for thy teeth and gums daily and see thy dentist and hygienist every six months.

8. Thou shalt monitor thy blood glucose levels on a regular basis and especially do a test when thou does not want to.

9. Thou shalt check thy feet daily and see a podiatrist every two to three months.

10. Thou shalt wear thy medical ID tag now and forever.

11. Thou shalt not smoke nor take up any tobacco products.

12. Thou shalt get a flu shot every year and thou shalt wear thy seat belt at all times whither thou goest.

13. If thou art woman and thy womb be fertile, thou shalt remember that bad blood sugars beget big bad babies with health problems. Do not beget any babies until thy blood sugars art in perfect control and thy doctor hath blessed any begettin'.

14. Thou shalt do something every day in the way of a healthy and pleasurable activity for thy body, thy mind, and thy spirit.

15. Thou shalt love thyself as a worthwhile person with many wonderful qualities and facets and not flog thyself for having diabetes or for the occasional blooper blood glucose.

Amen

REFERENCE SECTION

A Few of Our Favorite Things

BEFORE WE SIGN OFF, WE WANT TO LEAVE YOU A FEW LITTLE somethings to remember us by and to help you stay on the path of diabetes virtue. We have found these healthful, helpful, and even entertaining over time, and we hope they will do the same for you.

Throughout this book we've suggested that you get yourself a computer or use one at your local public library so you can check out various Web sites for the latest diabetes information.

We say it again.

But we also want to deliver to you a big BEWARE—not all Web sites are created equal. When you're browsing and pondering the information on these sites, you must remember an old saying: "If it sounds too good to be true, it probably is." (The same holds true if it sounds too bad. Could it be that they're using scare tactics to convince you to purchase a product or subscribe to a service?) An even more important thing to remember is to "consider the source." Is the individual or organization putting forth the information reputable? Have you ever heard of them? Are they recognized in the wonderful world of diabetes therapy? Do they list people and/or organizations on their site that you *have* heard of and over the years have come to respect?

But before we get onto the Internet, we want to give our animal caregivers their due.

A *Cat*-alyst for your health

As you've read on page 261, heart attacks are high on the list of potential risk factors for people with diabetes, and we should do everything possible to prevent them. Along with the conventional methods of avoidance, we offer: cats. Cats?! Yes, cats. Although we have two of these fur-covered disease deflectors, this is not our idea, but that of Dr. Adnan Qureshi, executive director of the Minnesota Stroke Institute. According to him, owning a cat may lower your risk of dying from a heart attack. Statistically, non–cat owners have a 40 percent higher risk of dying from myocardial infarction than cat owners. This intelligence was based on the data of 4,435 people from the second National Health and Nutrition Examination Survey.

Dr. Qureshi admits that there isn't enough evidence to recommend getting a cat as a standard preventive therapy, but on the other hand, "unlike other medical interventions, which have a risk and a cost associated with it, this has minimal risk and isn't as costly. There's not much harm to it."

Well, how about dogs? What can they do for you? Let's give them equal time:

Dogs 4Diabetics
www.dogs4diabetics.com

If you found cats preventing heart attacks hard to believe, wait until you hear this: **Dogs 4Diabetics** is a nonprofit organization that trains dogs to identify and, more important, act upon the subtle scent changes that hypoglycemia (low blood glucose) creates in body chemistry, changes that are undetectable to their human companions. The Web site contains success stories, news, and events. The following story from the site will give you an idea of what a medical alert assistance dog can do for a person with diabetes:

Crystal and "Dela"

Life with diabetes is exhausting, and life with diabetes in a nondiabetic family and circle of friends is sometimes lonely. Dela changed that for me. Dela is my medical alert service dog that I received from Dogs 4 Diabetics a year and a half ago. It is difficult for me to put into words what Dela has done for me. I have had type 1 diabetes for fourteen years, and when I was first diagnosed, I felt like my life was over. Early on, I was told that having diabetes is like having a permanent part-time job from which I can never take time off. Now with Dela, I can at least share the work of catching hypoglycemic episodes. Dela is always working and always right. The best part for me is that when she helps me, it's nonjudgmental. She is my constant companion.

Take a look at this Web site. You will find it fascinating, and even if you don't need a Dela for yourself, you may know someone who does. Pass it on!

Children With Diabetes
www.childrenwithdiabetes.com

Back in 1995, the Web site **Children With Diabetes** was launched with the goals of helping the then-two-year-old Marissa Hitchcock meet other kids who had diabetes and of sharing the experiences of her parents, Jeff and Brenda. Before they knew what was happening, the site grew into the valuable and influential resource that it is today, with national conferences and events. In the beginning, the site was aimed primarily at type 1 children, but now, because of burgeoning growth and changing needs in diabetes, it has morphed into "the online community for kids, families, and adults with diabetes" of today. And, yes, that includes type 2s.

DiabetesSisters
www.diabetessisters.com

Did you ever wish you had a sister you could talk to frankly about your diabetes? Someone knowledgeable and compassionate who could understand what you're going through? Well, actually, you do: Brandy Barnes, the founder and editor of **Diabetes Sisters**. She was diagnosed with diabetes at the age of fifteen. Her "insatiable thirst for knowledge" and curiosity was further piqued by this diagnosis. In college at UNC Chapel Hill, she majored in psychology to feed her interest in "the human mind and how we train ourselves to overcome obstacles in life," and later went to graduate school at UNC School of Social Work. One thing led to another, culminating in the founding of the Diabetes Sisters Web site.

There, you will not only find information on an array of topics such as pregnancy, menopause, and adoption, but also an international and interactive community—there are blogs, message boards, and you can post comments on every one. Brandy's ultimate goal is to "capture the voice of all women with diabetes through the Diabetes Sisters Web site." Let your voice be captured!

David Mendosa
www.mendosa.com

Several years ago, we had the good fortune to be involved with a diabetes Web site where we became acquainted with David Mendosa, a man of many interests and talents, especially when it comes to diabetes. On his site, he verbally tackles every aspect of the condition and brings it down to earth. His has been rightly called "one of the most comprehensive and eclectic diabetes sites on the Web." Just glancing at the headings (food, exercise, medication, meters, complications, and advice for newbies) will give you an idea—but only an idea—of the manifold subjects covered. P.S. Don't miss the updating newsletter at the end of every issue.

David makes no profit from his Web site. It's a labor of love. As he says: "It's a way to give back to the Internet what the Internet gave me." Actually, it should be what the Internet took from him. In his biography (included on the site) he explains that before his diagnosis and concomitant enlightenment, he weighed three hundred pounds. Now, as you will see from his handsome, outdoorsy picture on the site, those days are gone.

Diabetes Mall
www.diabetesnet.com/ishop/

This site is owned by John Walsh and his wife, Ruth Roberts. John is a diabetes clinical specialist who has had diabetes for forty-eight years, and Ruth is a respected educator and medical writer. They are both knowledgeable and personally concerned with getting the best and most up-to-date information out to those folks in the diabetes community. Their wide selection of books—most at money-saving prices—along with a selection of diabetes-related products, are described in their catalog and on their site (in English, Spanish, and German).

The Diabetes Mall, 1030 W. Upas Street, San Diego, CA 92103; Phone: 1-800-988-4772; Fax: 1-619-497-0900

The American Diabetes Association (ADA)
www.diabetes.org

Established in 1940, the organization has been working ever since to "prevent and cure diabetes and improve the lives of all people with diabetes." Not surprisingly, after all those years of work, the ADA has got it right yet still manages to keep getting it better.

To learn about all the facets of the operation, go to the Web site. There you can find out how to join up and partake of many benefits, including a subscription to *Diabetes Forecast* (the ADA's monthly magazine), which is excellent. You also get a discount on the many books and diabetes products offered.

Surgical Weight-Loss Options

Bariatric Surgery for Obesity

Surgical weight-loss options have become increasingly popular, especially since a number of celebrities have undergone this option—for example Al Roker on the *Today* show. Many insurance companies pay for these procedures, although in my region, insurance companies are more often writing the policy with exclusions for any weight-loss surgery. To qualify, most insurance companies require that a person have a body mass index greater than 40, or over 35 with comorbidities (diabetes, hypertension, sleep apnea, arthritis). You can find out your body mass index by checking the chart on page 134.

There are several types of restrictive and combined restrictive and malabsorptive operations. Each has its own benefits and risks.

Restrictive Operations

Purely restrictive operations only limit food intake and do not interfere with the normal digestive process. To perform this operation, doctors create a small pouch at the top of the stomach where food enters from the esophagus. At first, the pouch holds about one ounce of food and later may stretch to two to three ounces. The lower outlet of the pouch is usually about a half inch in diameter or smaller. This small outlet delays the emptying of food from the pouch into the larger part of the stomach and causes a feeling of fullness.

After the operation, patients can no longer eat large amounts of food at one time. Most patients can eat about one-half to one cup of food without discomfort or nausea, but the food has to be soft, moist, and well chewed. Patients who undergo restrictive procedures generally are not able to eat as much as those who have combined operations.

Adjustable Gastric Banding

Purely restrictive operations for obesity include adjustable gastric banding (AGB), also called the "lap band" because it can be done by laparoscopy and is therefore often done in an outpatient setting.

In this procedure, a hollow band made of silicone rubber is placed around the stomach near its upper end, creating a small pouch and a narrow passage into the rest of the stomach. The band is then inflated with a salt solution through a tube that connects the band to an access port placed under the skin. It can be tightened or loosened over time to change the size of the passage by increasing or decreasing the amount of salt solution.

ADVANTAGES: Restrictive operations are easier to perform and are generally safer than malabsorptive operations. AGB is usually done via laparoscopy, which uses smaller incisions, creates less tissue damage, and involves shorter operating time and hospital stays than open procedures. Restrictive operations can be reversed if necessary, and result in few nutritional deficiencies. Laparoscopic surgery is a procedure done with the assistance of a very small video camera and very thin instruments through small incisions, about 1/2 inch.

DISADVANTAGES: Patients who undergo restrictive operations generally lose less weight than patients who have malabsorptive operations, and are less likely to maintain weight loss over the long term. Patients generally lose about half of their excess body weight in the first year after restrictive procedures. Some patients regain weight by eating high-calorie soft foods that easily pass through the opening to the stomach. Others are unable to change their eating habits and do not lose much weight to begin with. Successful results depend on the patient's willingness to adopt a long-term plan of healthy eating and regular physical activity.

RISKS: One of the most common risks of restrictive operations is vomiting, which occurs when the patient eats too much or the narrow passage into the larger part of the stomach is blocked. Another is slippage or wearing away of the band. A common risk of AGB is breaks in the tubing between the band and the access port. This can cause the salt solution to leak, requiring another operation to repair. Some patients experience infections and bleeding, but this is much less common than other risks. Although restrictive operations are the safest of the bariatric procedures, they still carry risk—in less than 1 percent of all cases, complications can result in death.

Because combined operations result in greater weight loss than restrictive operations, they may also be more effective in improving the health problems associated with severe obesity, such as hypertension (high blood pressure), sleep apnea, type 2 diabetes, and osteoarthritis.

Combined Restrictive/Malabsorptive Operations

Combined operations are the most common bariatric procedures. They restrict both food intake and the amount of calories and nutrients the body absorbs.

Roux-en-Y Gastric Bypass (RGB)

This operation is the most common and successful combined procedure in the United States. First, the surgeon creates a small stomach pouch to restrict food intake. Next, a Y-shaped section of the small intestine is attached to the pouch to allow food to bypass the lower stomach, the duodenum (the first segment of the small intestine), and the first portion of the jejunum (the second segment of the small intestine). This reduces the amount of calories and nutrients the body absorbs. Rarely, a cholecystectomy (gallbladder removal) is performed to avoid the gallstones that may result from rapid weight loss. More commonly, patients take medication after the operation to dissolve gallstones.

RECOMMENDED READING

Countdown, the magazine of the Juvenile Diabetes Foundation International, 432 Park Avenue South, New York, NY 10016-8013 (1-800-223-1138). Published four times a year. Subscription price $25.

Diabetes Dateline, a publication of the National Diabetes Information Clearinghouse (NDIC), Bethesda, MD 20892-3560 (1-301-654-3327). Meant primarily for professionals but also contains up-to-date information of value to the population of people with diabetes. Published two or three times a year. Subscription is free.

Diabetes Forecast, the magazine of the American Diabetes Association, 1660 Duke Street, Alexandria, VA 22314 (1-800-232-3472). Published monthly. Membership dues are $24 per year, $10 of which is designated for the subscription.

Diabetes Interview, 3715 Balboa Street, San Francisco, CA 94121 (1-800-488-8468). A consumer-oriented newspaper for the diabetes community; includes reports on current research, business briefs, articles. Published monthly. Subscription price $14.

Diabetes Self-Management, P.O. Box 52890, Boulder, CO 80322-2890 (1-800-234-0923). A distinguished board of contributing editors provides articles of special usefulness for diabetes self-care. Published bimonthly. Subscription price $18.

DIABETES WEB SITES

There are few things growing as fast as the number of health Web sites on the Internet, and their quality varies from excellent to worthless and/or dangerous. The following diabetes-related sites are recommended as excellent online resources:

American Association of Diabetes Educators
www.diabeteseducator.org

American Diabetes Association
www.diabetes.org

American Podiatric Medical Association
www.apma.org

Centers for Disease Control and Prevention
www.cdc.gov/diabetes

Juvenile Diabetes Research Foundation International
www.jdrf.org

Diabetes Action Research and Education Foundation
www.daref.org

Diabetes News Index
www.onhealth.com

Diabetes Prevention Program
diabetes.niddk.nih.gov/dm/pubs/preventionprogram/

Index

ABOUT THE AUTHORS

VIRGINIA VALENTINE, CNS, BC-ADM, CDE, HAS BEEN HELPING people manage their diabetes for more than twenty-five years. She is currently the co-owner and CEO of Diabetes Network, Inc., an American Diabetes Association–recognized program. In 1999, Ms. Valentine was awarded the Roche/Zitter Diabetes Disease Management Award, and she is a past recipient of the Diabetes Educator of the Year Award and the 2006 recipient of the Distinguished Service Award from the American Association of Diabetes Educators.

Virginia received her master of science in nursing degree from the University of Oklahoma College of Nursing. She holds faculty appointments with both the University of New Mexico College of Nursing and School of Medicine. She is a member of the Advanced Practice Advisory Board to the New Mexico Board of Nursing and serves as past president of the New Mexico Leadership Council of the American Diabetes Association.

JUNE BIERMANN AND BARBARA TOOHEY are the authors of the best sellers *The Diabetic's Book* and *The Diabetic's Total Health and Happiness Book*, as well as *The Stroke Book* and seven other health books. They live in California.